BUILDING *on* OUR PROMISE

INDIANA UNIVERSITY PRESS

BUILDING *on* OUR PROMISE

A History of Indiana University Health Bloomington

BARB BERGGOETZ

This book is a publication of

Indiana University Press
Office of Scholarly Publishing
Herman B Wells Library 350
1320 East 10th Street
Bloomington, Indiana 47405 USA

iupress.org

This book is printed on acid-free paper.

Manufactured in Canada

First Printing 2021

ISBN 978-0-253-05917-8 (hdbk.)

*This beautiful book would not have been possible without
Sandy DeWeese. Indiana University Health thanks her for her passion
and effort to bring this project to fruition and also for her many years
of service dedicated to improving health care in our community.*

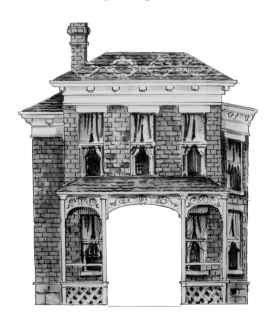

CONTENTS

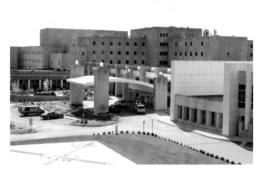

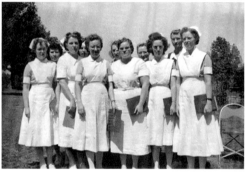

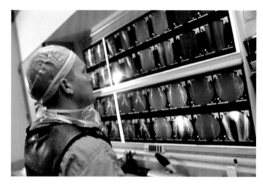

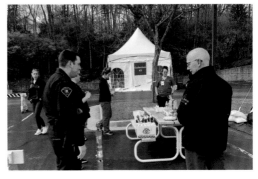

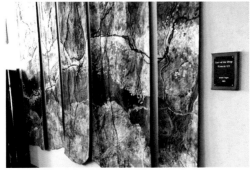

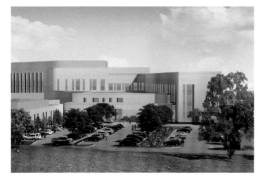

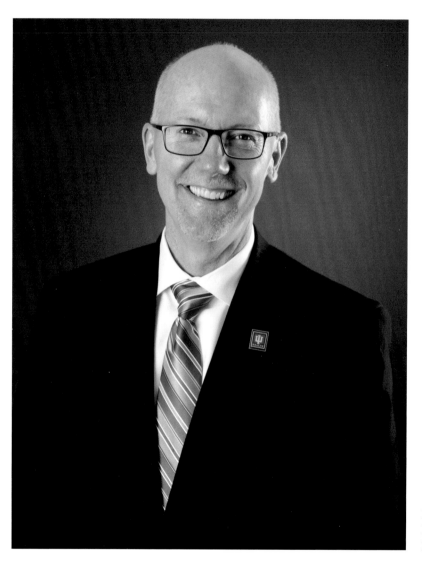

Brian Shockney, president and CEO of
IU Health South Central Region and
IU Health Bloomington Hospital

FOREWORD

Hospitals are about people—the people who live in the community, the people who care for the community. While advances in medical technology and new pharmaceuticals are most often in the spotlight, we remember every day that the human interaction of caring for each other defines health care in a way it does not define other industries. That is the story of Bloomington Hospital.

The women of Bloomington came together in 1905 to purchase property and convert a farmhouse into the first hospital building in Bloomington. Those strong women united around a common purpose and led the way for community development of health care services that would advance not just medical care but the economy and overall quality of life for an entire region. The values they represented continue today with the migration of IU Health Bloomington Hospital to a new location where it will continue to develop as a Regional Academic Health Center, serving eleven counties of south central Indiana.

As health care evolves, our services must as well. The new Regional Academic Health Center will start a new chapter, but we recognize the importance of building on our history and of celebrating the achievements of those who came before us. Well-designed buildings provide a resource critical to deliver care, but success and growth is possible only because of the strength of our hospital leaders and medical professionals, the involvement of our community, and the continued development of a team striving for excellent and compassionate care.

IU Heath Bloomington Hospital will work every day to deserve the trust of the community we serve. Thank you for celebrating with us, and I hope you enjoy this look back at our rich heritage and join us as we step into the future.

Brian T. Shockney
President, IU Health South Central Region

ACKNOWLEDGMENTS

I am very grateful for the advice and feedback from Sandy DeWeese, a long-time administrator and nurse for IU Health Bloomington Hospital, who guided me through writing this book, suggested the best people to interview, and provided encouragement and a deep understanding of the hospital's history. Brian Shockney, president and CEO of IU Health South Central Region, deserves credit for providing the vision for this special commemoration of the hospital.

I also am so appreciative of many doctors, nurses, hospital administrators, and board members, as well as community leaders and health care experts, who spent countless hours sharing their insights, opinions, and knowledge with me about the hospital's growth, impact, and importance to the community. The Monroe County History Center's files, including articles from the *Bloomington Herald-Times*, provided invaluable facts and background information. I especially enjoyed talking with patients and employees, whose heartfelt descriptions of the health care they received or provided brought to life the hospital's significance in the lives of many people.

Barb Berggoetz

BUILDING *on* OUR PROMISE

1

COMPASSION, GROWTH, AND MAKING BLOOMINGTON EVER HEALTHIER FOR 116 YEARS

FOR ALMOST A MONTH, Laura Balsmeyer lay in Bloomington Hospital's intensive care unit, at times, fighting for her life. She arrived in septic shock and underwent emergency surgery on her intestines—then another surgery. Her condition was bleak. But in time, she pulled through.

Both she and her husband Brian Balsmeyer, football coach at Paoli High School at the time, said they were overwhelmed by the quality of her care, the attention, patience, and kindness of her doctor, nurses, pharmacist, and everyone who cared for her and supported the family. The Balsmeyers felt so grateful they invited their 12 "Game Changers" to one of his games, where the medical team was publicly recognized on the field and in a hospitality tent.

Two years later, she had a heart attack. Brian remembered thinking, "The people in Bloomington loved her so much so if these are going to be her last days, I want her to be at Bloomington Hospital."

Again, she survived.

"Those people have a special place in our hearts," he said. "What a blessing they were to us."

❧❧

While talking on the phone with a Chicago business associate, lifelong Bloomington resident Fred Dunn suddenly dropped the phone. At age 65, Dunn had no serious health issues. He doesn't

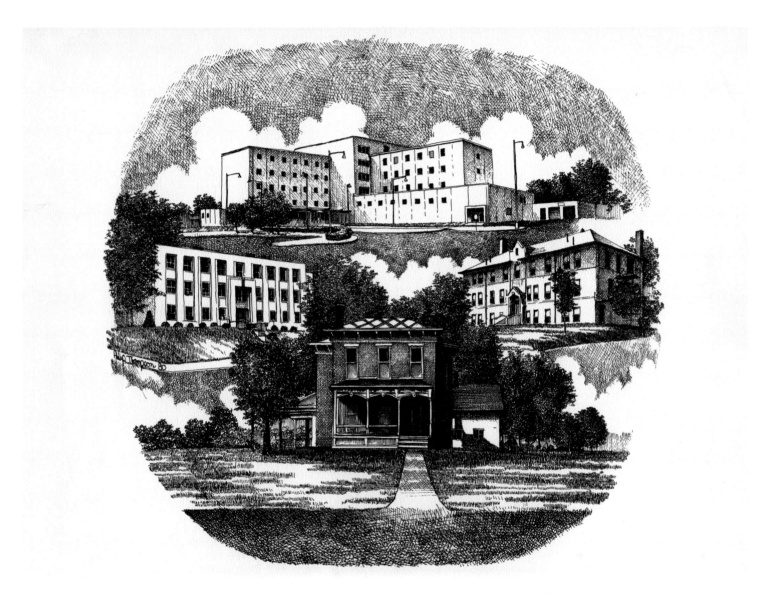

Pen-and-ink collage sketch of four buildings of Bloomington Hospital.
This is a print of a drawing done by Phillip Thompson in 1980. *Photo
credit: Monroe County History Center Collection, Bloomington, Indiana.*

remember much about the incident, but he knew something was wrong. His speech was slurred. He was weak.

Dunn had suffered a major stroke. Luckily, his associate called a friend in Bloomington, and Dunn's brother, a doctor, was contacted and quickly got him to Bloomington Hospital. Dunn had lost some function in his left arm and leg, causing balance and coordination problems.

"The hospital was fantastic," he said. "Getting there in time and getting their protocol and help prevented the real damage from happening." Physical therapy helped him recover almost completely. He's benefited greatly from the hospital's stroke survivors' group, too. Guest speakers have helped him better understand strokes and learn about medicines and diet. And he's enjoyed sharing stories with others who've had strokes.

"It's great community outreach," said Dunn, now 77. "It's just a marvelous program."

More than 31 years ago, Paula Rice and a group of about 30 other employees were asked by hospital President Roland "Bud" Kohr to divide into pairs during an orientation program in the Medical Arts Building basement, which was under renovation. One person in each pair, she vividly recalled, put on a blindfold and the other led the person by hand around sawhorses and pipes, up a stairwell, outside and back inside, and downstairs again.

No one really knew why they were doing this, said Rice, an assistant in the behavioral health unit. But soon the purpose of the "Bud Kohr walk-thru" was quite clear.

"He wanted us to realize the responsibility we all had to patients," Rice remembered. "This was a lesson in putting yourself in the patient's place—that we must take care to lead our patients into the unknown and help them build a trust with someone they have never met.

"I will never forget it," Rice said.

An ICU patient and her husband, a stroke victim, and a long-time hospital employee all were deeply impacted by their experiences at IU Health Bloomington Hospital in vastly different ways. But each memory shares a common theme—a compassionate, skilled staff and a hospital system that works to provide the best health care possible to its patients and the community at large.

Much brain power, perseverance, and foresight—starting with a group of Bloomington female leaders more than a century ago—have led to today's IU Health Bloomington Hospital moving to the new IU Health Regional Academic Health Center.

In its 116 years of existence, the hospital has grown from a tiny, independent community hospital, first owned and operated by the Local Council of Women, to become part of IU Health's statewide system in 2010. In countless ways, the hospital has thrived, along with Bloomington and Indiana University, and improved and expanded its medical practices, health care delivery, and accessibility.

As the largest and most comprehensive health care facility between Indianapolis and Louisville, Bloomington Hospital, now expanded to a 24-acre campus, is regionally recognized for specialized cardiac, obstetrics, and emergency services, as well as its skilled care in oncology, orthopedics, psychiatry, diabetes, and more.

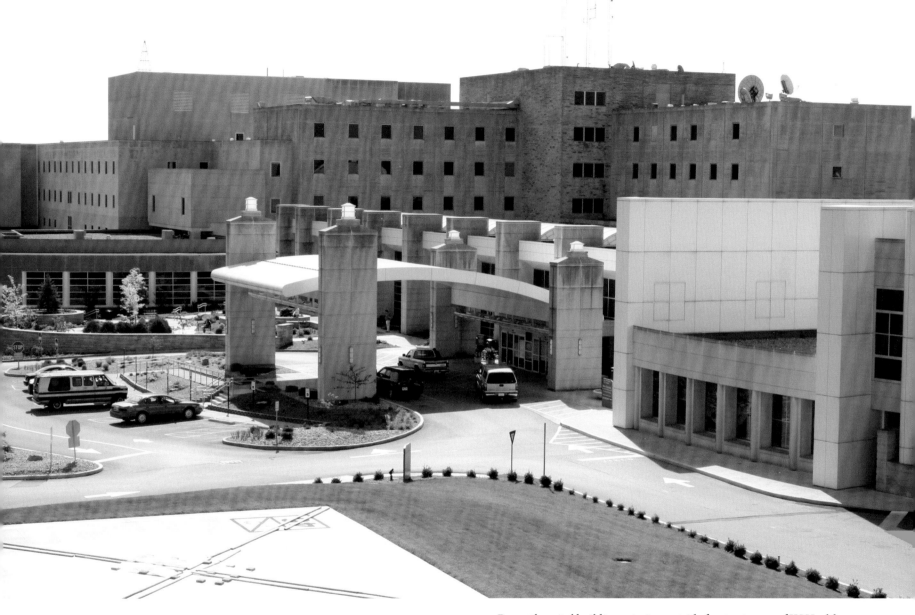

Recent hospital building exterior: outside front entrance of IU Health
Bloomington Hospital. *Photo credit: IU Health Bloomington Hospital.*

Over those years, hospital administrators, in concert with local physicians and medical specialists, nurses, community health staff, and local business leaders alike, have pushed and pulled each other to adopt medical advances, create up-to-date facilities, pursue modern technology, and provide services to meet the health needs of the community.

It wasn't always easy. And it wasn't always seamless. Hundreds of millions of dollars had to be raised and borrowed. Controversies emerged. Debates arose in the community and among doctors and administrators over the best path forward.

But issues were eventually settled.

Changes, advances, discoveries were made. New services were developed to keep up with demands. Efficiencies were found. Health crises on individual and community-wide levels were encountered and dealt with over and over. On many fronts, health care improved.

Always, progress resulted. Along the way, the community's health care needs were largely met, agreed many health care and community leaders interviewed for this book.

Bloomington Hospital played an oversized role in all of this.

"We're the engine that has the resources," said Brian Shockney, CEO and president of IU Health South Central Indiana since November 2016 and a hospital administrator for 35 years. "Physicians are the highly trained scientists."

The hospital serves as the link binding the system together, said Jefferson Shreve, former hospital board of directors member, local business owner, and volunteer leader.

"I would describe it as the central connector to a health care system in the community. A hospital system is part of the connective tissue of the health care ecosystem," said Shreve, president

and owner of Storage Express, a five-state business. "You can have smaller or underserved communities who have practitioners, but they tend to be generalists, rather than specialists. The specialists need to be able to apply their craft as credentialed physicians at a hospital because that's where they do their work," said Shreve, who served for two hospital board terms as a representative of the Local Council of Women.

"You apply your craft at a hospital with surgical wards, and critical care units, and in-patients. So the hospital, as a central part of the health care system, is at the center of that web of health care delivery in the community," he said.

The hospital's physical facilities have monumentally changed and expanded since that first two-story, red brick building at South Rogers and First Streets was converted into a 10-bed hospital in 1905. That was the work of female leaders who little could have realized the ultimate results of the health care crusade they put in motion. They were moved to do so by a tragic 1904 train accident that killed a man in Bloomington who needed more extensive medical care than was available then.

Today, IU Health Bloomington Hospital serves a population base of more than 467,600 in an 11-county area from Morgan County down to Washington and Orange Counties. With a highly skilled medical staff of 484 physicians practicing 43 medical specialties, the hospital offers a wide range of services using state-of-the-art technology, creative innovations, and collaborative partnerships while benefiting from ongoing community support.

The physicians, nurses, technicians, social service staff, and many others in the 337-bed hospital perform critical work in a fast-paced environment changing every day to meet patients' and community needs, even under the unprecedented challenges presented by the COVID-19 pandemic that began in early 2020.

"I have been a part of several significant events that stressed hospital resources for a short period of time in my career, but nothing like this," said Shockney. "I have never experienced such incredible dedication to our mission and most likely never will in the remainder of my career."

Health care leaders, he explained, train throughout their careers for natural disasters and pandemics through emergency preparedness programs. "Therefore, we had the tools, processes and structures in place to immediately begin to address the spread of the virus in our region and care for all patients who needed care."

But he said COVID-19 presented particularly tough challenges that the hospital met head-on.

"This virus was very new to the world and, similar to the HIV/AIDS virus when I was in college, we had to quickly discover and learn ongoing about its epidemiology," Shockney stressed. "Our team members chose health care as their calling because they seek to do good in the lives of others. This value and passion kicked into overdrive with the pandemic and our team of physicians, providers, nurses, technicians, support personnel and leaders gave their all to ensuring the best care at every opportunity."

The typical day-to-day events at the hospital—surgeries, births, emergencies, outpatient care—may not present the same daunting challenges. But, clearly, health care providers face demanding tasks each time they walk through the hospital doors.

As of 2019, Bloomington Hospital admitted 14,176 patients, who stayed an average of 4.4 days. Babies are born every day—a total of 1,737 that year. The emergency department treated 52,378

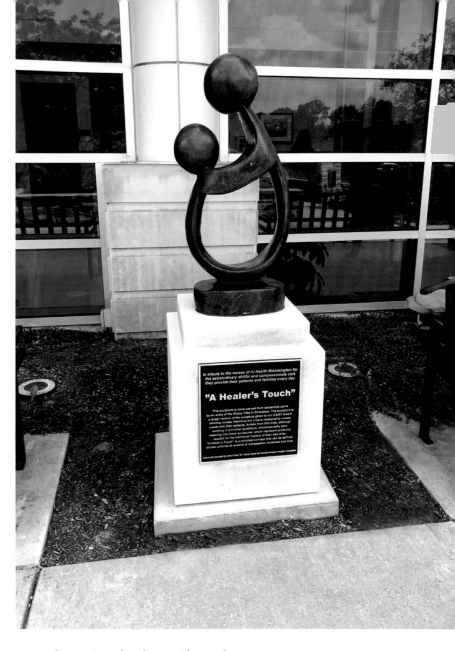

Hospital Daisy Award sculpture at hospital.
Photo credit: IU Health Bloomington Hospital.

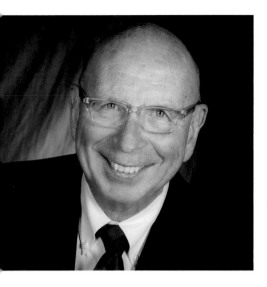

people seeking immediate medical care. And more than 8,900 outpatient surgery visits and nearly 3,350 inpatient surgery visits occurred throughout the year.[1]

But numbers just give a glimpse of all that goes on every day within the hospital's walls. They don't tell the stories of patients like Balsmeyer and Dunn and staff member Rice, all of whom are portrayed more fully later in this book.

To commemorate the hospital's legacy as it moves into the IU Health Regional Academic Health Center, the book retraces its history, physical development, and medical and technological advancements. The book also describes the overall impact and significance of the hospital in the community, through the eyes of hospital, community, and business leaders. In addition, the book highlights health care leaders and providers who contributed to the hospital's growth and some patients who received that care.

In the eyes of Lynn Coyne, a community and business leader and chairman of the final IU Health Bloomington Hospital board

Above, Lynn Coyne, attorney of counsel with Bunger and Robertson and long-time community leader, is a member of the IU Health South Central Region board of directors and past chairman of the IU Health Bloomington Hospital board. *Photo submitted by Lynn Coyne.*

of directors, the hospital has been an integral part of what makes this unique city an attractive and safe place to live.

"You want to be in Bloomington because it has a great hospital, lots of doctors, a university, and a lot of culture," said Coyne, an attorney of counsel with Bunger and Robertson. "It is now a co-equal component of a vibrant community. It's no longer a small, antiquated facility. It's matching what we need to grow."

With 2,352 employees, the hospital is the third-largest employer in Bloomington, behind IU and Cook Group. Coyne, former president and past board chairman of the Bloomington Economic Development Corporation, said the hospital actually provides good stable employment for the region.

"It is, in and of itself, an economic engine," said Coyne, who now sits on the IU Health South Central Region Board of Directors. "It hires people. It creates jobs. It creates services to support a community that makes it the kind of community you want to be in."

From a little different vantage point, Ken G. Stella has watched Bloomington Hospital progress over the years while he was president of the Indiana Hospital Association from 1994 to 2007.

"It was able to stay independent quite a while," Stella observed, while noting that many other Indiana independent hospitals merged sooner or didn't survive. "Bloomington Hospital had a hell of an advantage because of the city and university. People wanted to live there, and young doctors loved to come to Bloomington."

Because of those advantages, Stella added, the hospital "always had an excellent medical staff." On the other hand, other communities had to work hard to recruit doctors, he said.

The Bloomington Hospital continued to grow and attract young doctors who were specialists in a variety of medical fields and who brought patients with them from surrounding counties, Stella explained. As a result, he said the hospital responded with resources to support programs and expanded facilities that doctors wanted. "That's how it became regional, because of the medical staff and continuing to get more and more specialists."

Local physicians who worked with the hospital and sometimes for the hospital recognized this symbiotic relationship, although some doctors also acknowledged that wasn't always the case during the hospital's history. Often, though, the partnerships were formed out of necessity.

"Everything is expensive, and so partnering with the hospital and its resources and the doctors and their talents allows us to merge the two together to provide better care," said Dr. James Laughlin, long-time pediatrician who now serves as chief practice officer of IU Health Bloomington Hospital.

"You've got the doctors and the hospital administrators working as a team, instead of in competition, to decide what equipment we need, what services we can provide, what the limits are of what we can do," explained Laughlin, who is a member of Southern Indiana Physicians. "Ideally, that's the reason we should be together."

Compared to other similar-size cities in Indiana, Laughlin also recognized Bloomington has had a fairly long tradition of having rather good specialty care available to residents.

But he also stressed another positive factor highlighting the hospital's history that has had a significant impact on the community over the years.

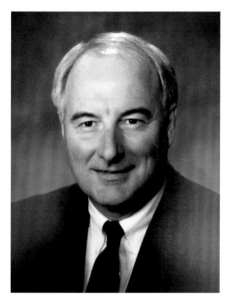

The region, largely to the hospital's credit, has been proud of being very proactive in providing resources for community health initiatives, he said. "We have a whole community health department in the hospital, which serves outpatient care for immunization, public health clinic needs, such as food stamp program, (baby) formula, and the WIC (Women, Infants and Children) counseling services for behavioral health. We have a whole program that provides addiction services for the community and the region."

Retired internist, Dr. Jean Creek, 92, acknowledged the major strides Bloomington Hospital has made and the positive effect it has had on the health and welfare of the community, particularly in the last half-century.

"It obviously had a big impact," said Creek, who started as a family practice physician here in 1955, became an internist, and also directed the hospital's medical education for 35 years. "I'm not giving myself credit for this, because there were a hell of a lot

Above, Ken G. Stella, now retired, has watched Bloomington Hospital progress over the years while he was president of the Indiana Hospital Association from 1994 to 2007. *Photo submitted by Ken Stella.*

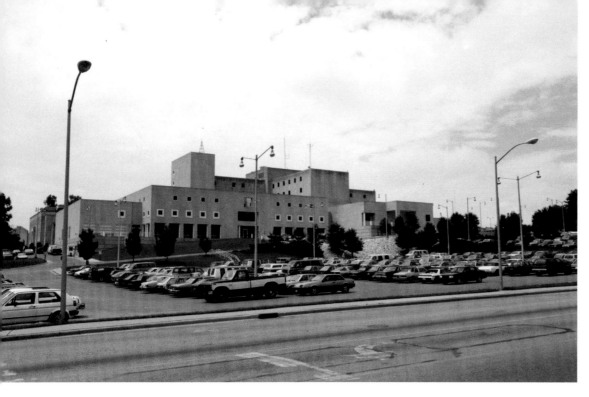

antismoking campaign; the leadership of hospital administrator Roland "Bud" Kohr; and hospital pathologist Dr. Tony Pizzo's teaching and behind-the-scenes influences on the hospital's operation.

The list of the hospital's accomplishments, milestones, and major players, inside and outside of the hospital, since 1905 is much longer and far-reaching. Many major donors, board of directors members, and local movers and shakers—not the least of whom is the late Bill Cook, founder of Cook Group. He was instrumental in funding the hospital's cardiac rehab program and catheterization lab and played substantial roles in increasing the hospital's stature and enhancing its impact.

of people who did it, but from the time I came here, which is all I can speak about, the hospital has improved 300%."

However, Creek recognized the hospital wasn't as proactive and progressive as other hospitals in similar-sized cities in the mid-century period until its board of directors changed and new administrators came on board. "Once we caught back up in the 1970s and early 1980s, I think we've been a very progressive hospital. I think a lot of it had to do with having a medical school here. This, in turn, brought in physicians who had specialties."

Many other changes, he said, led to the hospital's increasing stature: more authority given to nurses; medical education improvements; increased education of patients; additional social services provided patients; public health initiatives, such as the

As Bloomington Hospital leaves its long-time west Second Street home and begins a new life at the $557 million Regional Academic Health Center on the Indiana Route 45/46 bypass, health care providers, employees, and the community applaud this momentous move. But it's also worthwhile to look back at the people, key decisions, hard work, and compassionate care that created this distinguished regional hospital.

Above, Bloomington Hospital exterior view from Second Street before parking garage was added (date unknown). *Photo credit: Monroe County History Center Photo Collection, Bloomington, Indiana.*

Facing, Aerial photos of Regional Health Academic Center under construction in 2020. *Photo credit: IU Health Bloomington Hospital.*

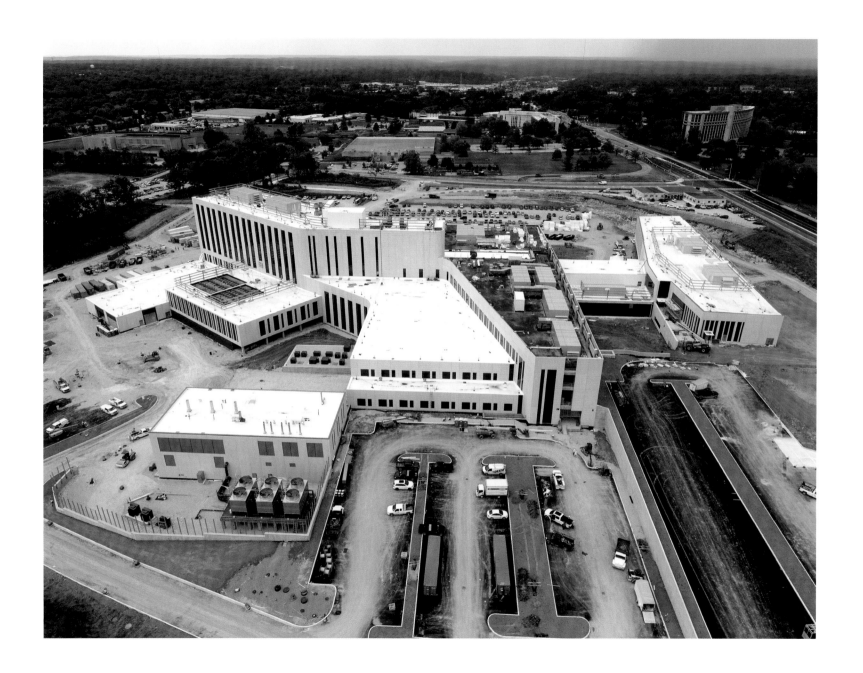

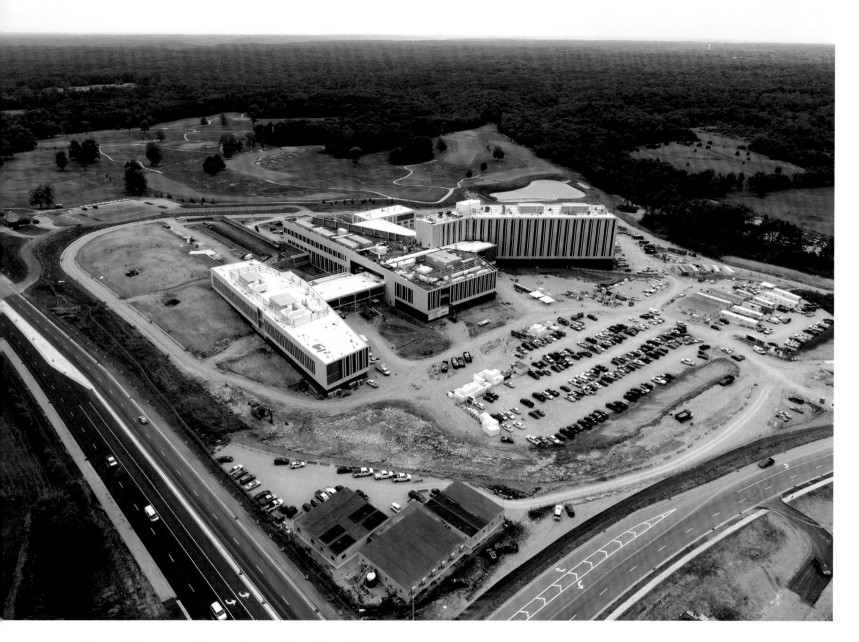

Above and facing, Aerial photos of Regional Health Academic Center under construction in 2020. *Photo credit: IU Health Bloomington Hospital.*

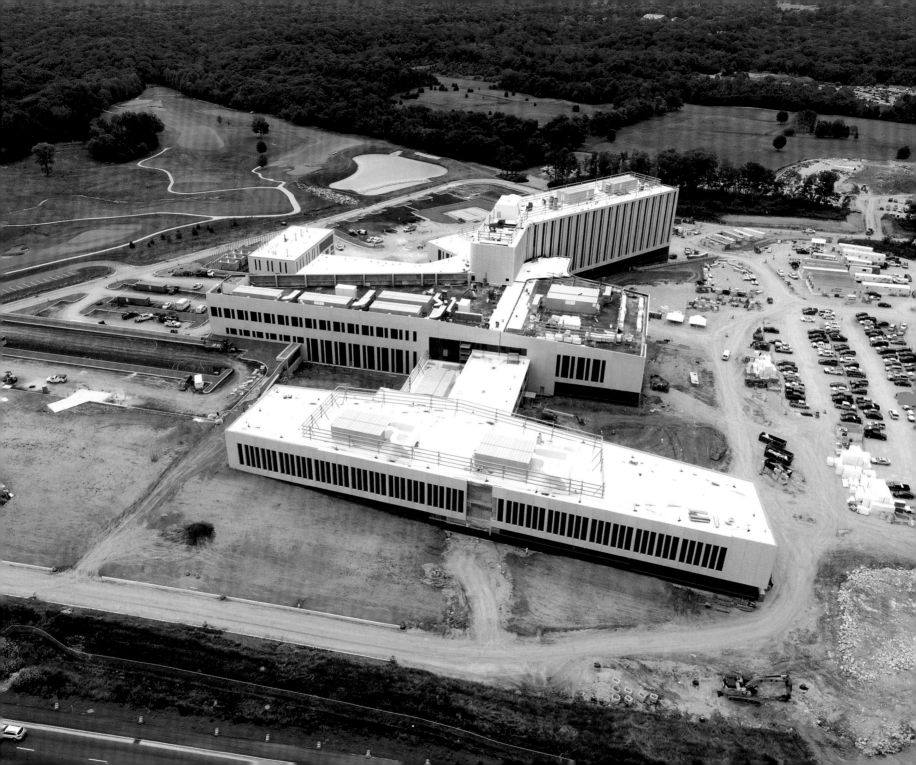

2

LOCAL COUNCIL OF WOMEN: DREAMERS, LEADERS, AND FUND-RAISERS

THE ROOTS OF BLOOMINGTON HOSPITAL are embedded in an outpouring of empathy and concern by local women and community members who realized in the early 1900s that their small town of 8,000 sorely needed a hospital to treat the sick, poor and all residents.

Female leaders from 17 diverse groups had banded together in 1897 to form the Local Council of Women, which still exists today. The council, comprising representatives from women's clubs devoted to literary, musical, civic, and philanthropic interests, was focused on improving their city and especially health care.[1] But a tragic train accident in late 1904 sparked their efforts.

The death of Lawrence Mitts, 32, who was crushed by a train near Bloomington in 1904 and later died, triggered the events leading to establishing the city's first hospital. Most accounts say Mitts had been working in Bloomington and was on his way home to visit his mother in New Albany when was found on the Monon railroad tracks on October 30, 1904. He'd apparently fallen asleep on the tracks and had been run over by a train, which badly mangled both of his legs. He was brought to the home of Dr. J. E. Harris, a local physician. Harris, his wife, and two other doctors worked through the night to try to save his life.[2] Unfortunately, their efforts were in vain.

Mitts was buried in Bloomington on November 1, 1904, as his family was too poor to bring him home and bury him, according to a lengthy hospital history written by Bea Snoddy, historian for the council and Bloomington Hospital. She wrote that Mrs. Harris, along with council representatives of the various clubs, met that night for their regular meeting at a local motor inn.[3]

But the meeting quickly took on a sense of urgency.

They recognized the immediate need, highlighted by the tragic accident, for Bloomington to have health care services available to handle such accidents and the needs of local residents. All voted in favor of pushing for a hospital, reported Snoddy. The vote followed a report from a council committee that had previously visited a Crawfordsville, Indiana, hospital that was funded in a similar manner as the women proposed the local hospital.

At the suggestion of Mrs. Harris, the council voted to secure the land and building, despite the challenge facing them. Snoddy quoted her as saying, "If Crawfordsville with a surplus of $60 to its treasury, can build a hospital, surely we can do as well with a surplus of $400."[4] Their resolve led to purchasing 4.5 acres of land with a 10-room red brick Italianate house on south Rogers Street between First and Second Streets.

"I would think it was very unusual back at the turn of the century because women couldn't even vote back then," said Susan Wier, a past council president and current member. "For these clubs to come together and raise the money to buy the hospital, I think it was very, very unusual.

"Even today, I'm impressed by them," stressed Weir, president and owner of First American Advisory LLC, a Bloomington registered investment advisory business. "It amazes me the determination they had and the way they all pulled together," added Wier, a former licensed practical nurse.

When the women formed the council, they wanted to unify their voices and concerns about issues in Bloomington, primarily related to health, such as the hazard of many horse and buggies tied up around the square downtown. At that time, roads were merely mud and dirt and the horses' wastes were polluting the area and draining onto streets during rainy weather, wrote council member Pat Bartlett in an address to the local Argonaut Club in April 2003.[5]

After the council was formed and incorporated, its mission statement demonstrated the breadth of members' concerns for numerous issues facing their small town. They were passionate about improving their families' living conditions and environment.

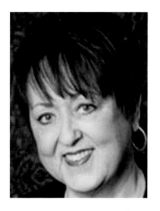

Susan Wier, a past Local Council of Women president and current member, is president and owner of First American Advisory LLC, a Bloomington registered investment advisory business. *Photo submitted by Susan Wier.*

The mission statement read: "Believing that the more intimate knowledge of one another's work will result in larger mutual sympathy and greater unity of thought, and therefore in more effective action, certain associations of women in Bloomington interested in religion, philosophy, education, literature, art, and social reform have determined to organize a Local Council."

At first, improvements in the city took much of members' time, wrote former member Cecilia H. Wahl, who also served as chairperson of the Bloomington Hospital board of directors, in a council history written in October 1995. They worked to keep the city clean, take care of the poor, increase school standards, raise $1,000 toward construction of a new Indiana University Student

Building, and promote a new library in town with the Sorosis Club, wrote Wahl.[6]

The council had always been involved in different health issues in the community, particularly in health care education, explained Wier. While the women were concerned with other issues of the day, they were most troubled about the lack of a local hospital, even before the train accident.

Their empathy may have emanated from their roles in society at the time.

"I think women were really the health care providers in the family," reflected Wier. "When something that tragic happened, if they had just had a hospital to operate on this man back then, maybe he would have lived. That was a time when people were very compassionate. This was the role women played. They couldn't be doctors, but they were definitely the caregivers in the community."

Women weren't readily accepted into medical school back in that time period, Wier pointed out. "If it were me living back at that time, I would have thought, 'Oh, my gosh, what if it was my husband who got killed?' Then we would be on the charity line because women didn't work outside the home for the most part."

Some of the women's groups had individually discussed the need for a hospital previously, as had the Local Council of Women during its October meeting. At that time, the council members agreed to take the idea of a city hospital back to their clubs to get feedback. But before the next meeting occurred, the fateful accident spurred action.

"This was the catalyst," said Wier.

A detailed accounting of the beginning of the train accident and the beginning of the hospital was spelled out in "A Short

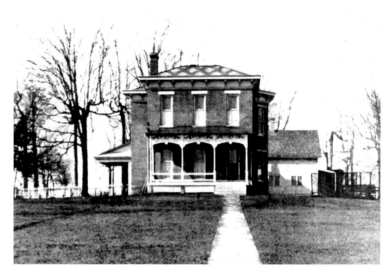

First home of Bloomington Hospital was a 10-room red brick farmhouse, purchased and renovated by the Local Council of Women and opened in 1905. *Photo credit: IU Health Bloomington Hospital.*

History of Bloomington Hospital," written on Oct. 8, 1951, by an unknown author. The director of that early council, assembled in the parlor of their president, discussed the accident in tears, the article reads. "Their determination was aroused. Bloomington should have a hospital," the article said.[7]

And they quickly got to work to make that happen.

The amount of money the council needed to raise for a hospital seems paltry now, yet it was a tall order for this newly formed group. It formally incorporated in February 1905 with 18 members and 11 directors. A committee was appointed to look for a location, and six men from the community were added. Three locations, including Dunn Meadow, a site in the northern portion of the county, and the Rogers Street property, were considered. After several meetings and much discussion, the council decided to purchase the Rogers Street property in December 1904 from a local man, Isaac P. Hopewell, even though it was $2,000 more expensive than the other sites. The new building was called the Hopewell House.[8]

The council was successful in raising $6,000 to buy the land and the red brick house, plus $3,000 for remodeling, according to an article in the April/May 2019 issue of the Monroe County Historian newsletter, written by Lee H. Ehman, a retired IU School of Education professor who volunteers for the Monroe County History Center Research Library.[9]

Cecilia H. Wahl, a former council member and chairperson of the Bloomington Hospital board of directors for three terms, wrote an article describing in detail the steps these women took to raise money. "How those ladies labored for the nickels, dimes and dollars! Rummage sale after rummage sale ($96 profit for the year), recitals, lectures, a theater benefit given by I.U.'s Strut and Fret Society; selling refreshments at the county fair, a baseball game, a hospital association with a minimum membership fee of $1 per year; donations of 12 dozen towels by Unique Club; donation of a 'real live cow,'" said Wahl in "The Women Behind the Local Council of Women," written in November 1989.

Wahl, a well-known community leader who was also secretary of the IU Board of Trustees in the 1960s, said council women also

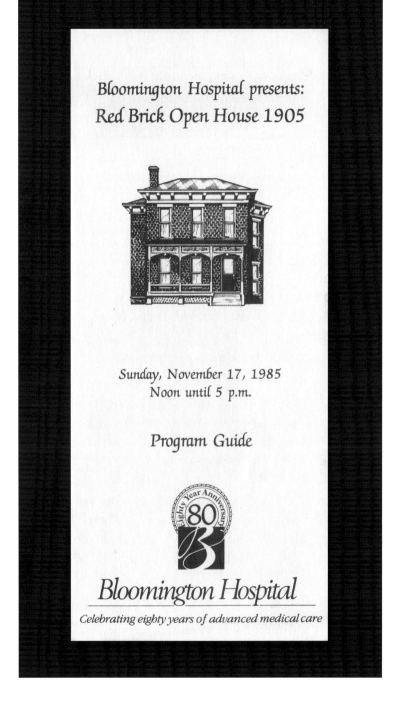

Illustration of program for Bloomington Hospital's Red Brick Open House on November 7, 1985, in recognition of hospital's first facility that opened in 1905. *Photo credit: Monroe County History Center Collection, Bloomington, Indiana.*

had traditional bake sales—anything to earn money from the community to pay for the building and furnish the hospital with the proper medical equipment, beds and linens.[10]

Their ideas eventually paid off, too.

"All these little bitty amounts of money that today would seem laughable, but back then they were major contributions," said Wier, a council member since 2000 who was council president in 2005 when Bloomington Hospital integrated with IU Health.

The house needed extensive remodeling to be suitable for a hospital. A steam heating plant was installed and plumbing added. Partitions in two large bedrooms upstairs created small, private rooms with a ward in the rear with three beds, designated for charity patients. The 10-bed hospital opened in November 1905, a year sooner than the women had thought possible because "the response, in money and furnishings, was liberal beyond all expectations," wrote Snoddy. Showers Brothers donated furniture, she said, and linens, bedding, and kitchen supplies were donated by local women's clubs.[11]

To meet growing expenses, council members continued to generate money in unique ways, including using local foodstuffs and even enlisting school children to contribute food. During World War I, council members also were asked to set aside one quart of fruit, vegetables, or jelly for the hospital.

"Part of the hospital's operating costs were met by the harvest from its garden and milk from the cow," wrote Snoddy. "School children were asked to bring a potato to class to be collected for the hospital larder. Each member organization of the Local Council of Women assumed responsibility for a room in the hospital and paid a room maintenance fee."[12]

On Thanksgiving Day that year, the hospital was formally dedicated—marking a major milestone in the development of Bloomington Hospital.

No patients were being treated that day, but the following day two patients were admitted, according to a brochure describing the hospital's history and philosophy, written by the Local Council of Women in October 1951. The brochure, stored at the Monroe County Public Library, said, "From one of these (patients), a professor from the neighboring Indiana University, a letter is preserved expressing his appreciation for hospital treatment during an appendicitis operation, and adding that his only regret was that he had but one appendix. This letter seems an omen of the friendly, informal spirit in which service was given and received by the hospital, a spirit which still persists."[13]

But hospital staff soon realized the building was not ideally configured for a hospital.

The operating room on the second floor was hard to reach, as the front stairway was steep, narrow, and winding. The back stairway, wrote Snoddy, was also unusable and was remodeled so that a stretcher could be carried up the stairs only by "heroic lifting and twisting on the part of the ambulance drivers, nurses and even the physician who was later to perform the operation."

Three nurses were hired to lead the hospital. Blanche Stoops, of Indianapolis, was superintendent, and Bessie Lemon and Mary Tague assisted her. They quickly started a training school for nurses. At first, the entire hospital staff actually lived in the hospital building, but as the number of patients increased, the council converted a woodshed on the property to a "nurses' home," wrote Snoddy. There, the nurses could rest without having to leave their beds at home for emergency patients.

Running a hospital, the women soon realized, required a different management structure. The Local Council of Women's officers recognized in 1906 that they should not be the sole members of the hospital's board of managers any longer. Instead, a 12-member hospital board was appointed, with staggered three-, two- and one-year terms, including five current council officers and seven other members elected from a slate of 10 other people.[14]

To properly staff the hospital, council leaders also soon realized they needed to train nurses. Beginning in 1906, the hospital conducted training its School of Practical Nursing, which continued until 1945 and resulted in graduating 124 nurses, according to the Monroe County Historian's April/May 2019 issue.[15]

Through all of the council members' hard work, the group was thrilled to be able to pay off all debt for the hospital and its equipment in early 1908. "It was a joyous occasion," wrote Snoddy. "That Bloomington had an adequate place to care for its sick was reward enough for the time and effort these women had expended during the preceding three years. While only 17 beds were available, including three kept for charity patients, the property was clear of debt and the women looked forward to finding ways and means of providing a bigger hospital."

But they knew their work wasn't done by any means. This was just the beginning.

While dedicated to providing health care to Bloomington residents, council women also recognized after five and a half years of operation that the hospital needed about six weeks in 1910

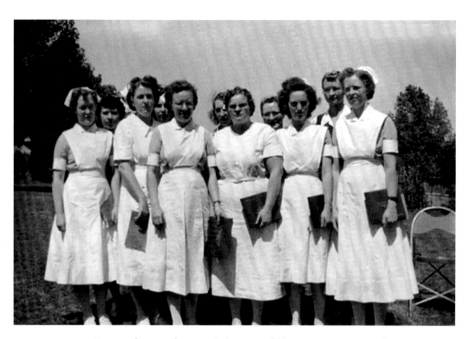

Group of nurses from early history of Bloomington Hospital (no further information available; photo from hospital centennial PowerPoint). *Photo credit: IU Health Bloomington Hospital.*

for a complete renovation. The women, according to Snoddy's report, made a detailed statement about the work done and the reasons the improvements, in order to bring further attention to the hospital's needs and finances. They said the hospital and nurses' cottage were completely cleaned, the walls and woodwork repainted and varnished, the roofs repaired, the furnace replaced, a bathroom added on the first floor, and a large private room created by changing a partition. They also said a wardroom was created on the second floor out of two small private rooms. So, the hospital had one ward for women and one for men.

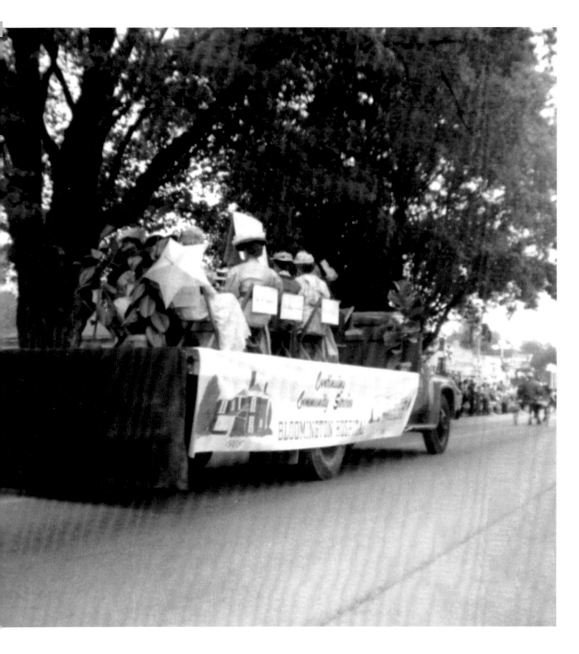

Bloomington Hospital parade float with women riding who are in period dress and who are possibly members of the Local Council of Women, which started the campaign for a Bloomington Hospital in 1904. *Photo credit: Monroe County History Center Photo Collection, Bloomington, Indiana.*

The council reported they had to borrow $5,000 to complete the work, on top of $2,000 previously borrowed for street and sewer assessments. In addition, the council women said the hospital superintendent has hired an experienced corps of nurses who have made the hospital a "much more efficient institution than it has ever been before, and is consequently more expensive to maintain," their statement said.

The goal expressed in their statement was a request to "friends of the hospital" to commit to contributing a certain amount for five years to create a "nurses fund." They appealed to "all the citizens of Bloomington to aid in removing the . . . debt, and in providing, each according to his means, a fund sufficient to maintain an institution which serves the rich and poor alike."[16]

The hospital's services were, indeed, being used by residents more and more. In 1914, for example, the *Bloomington Telephone* newspaper ran a "hospital report" for the last six months of that year, cited the Monroe County Historian's April/May 2019 issue. The report said the hospital served 98 patients, conducted 68 surgeries, and experienced three births and five deaths. Hospital earnings from fees totaled $2,000, while the city paid $300 and charities paid $200, leaving the facility with a $300 surplus.

Stressing rising numbers of patients, the council called for a larger building in the report, said the Monroe County Historian article.[17]

Council members and clubs affiliated continued to work hard to eliminate the hospital's debt from remodeling and rising operation costs. At the same time, though, they started focusing on their next goal—a new, larger hospital to better serve Bloomington.

Unfortunately, their first effort got sidetracked through no fault of their own.

The hospital board, consisting of council officers and other elected council members, hired an architect in April of 1917 to draw up plans for a new 35-bed limestone hospital to be built adjacent to the red brick building, Wahl explained. But the architect, Alfred Grindle of Indianapolis, suffered from health problems in 1918, and the plans couldn't be fully carried out at that time. But the foundation for the building had been laid at a cost of $2,200. Instead, the women concentrated on solving the financial difficulties of the current hospital, as well as raising funds for the new hospital.

By now, the United States had entered World War I, and many people were planting gardens to relieve food shortages. The council wanted to do its part, so it proposed all members contribute one quart of fruit, vegetables, or jelly for the hospital, Wahl wrote. This effort helped pay for higher costs of food, coal, drugs, and staff salaries without raising room prices.

It seemed, though, the older women of the community were doing most of the heavy lifting to bring in money. The idea that younger women needed to contribute more was brought up during an October 1917 meeting of the hospital board, Wahl noted in her article.

Board president, Mrs. J. B. Wilson, said, according to meeting minutes, "During this critical time in the life and history of our nation, the women must be sure to carry on two lines of work— that of caring for the people of our own community and the war relief work."

Council women responded to the board president's plea by renewing the campaign for a new hospital at their meeting in

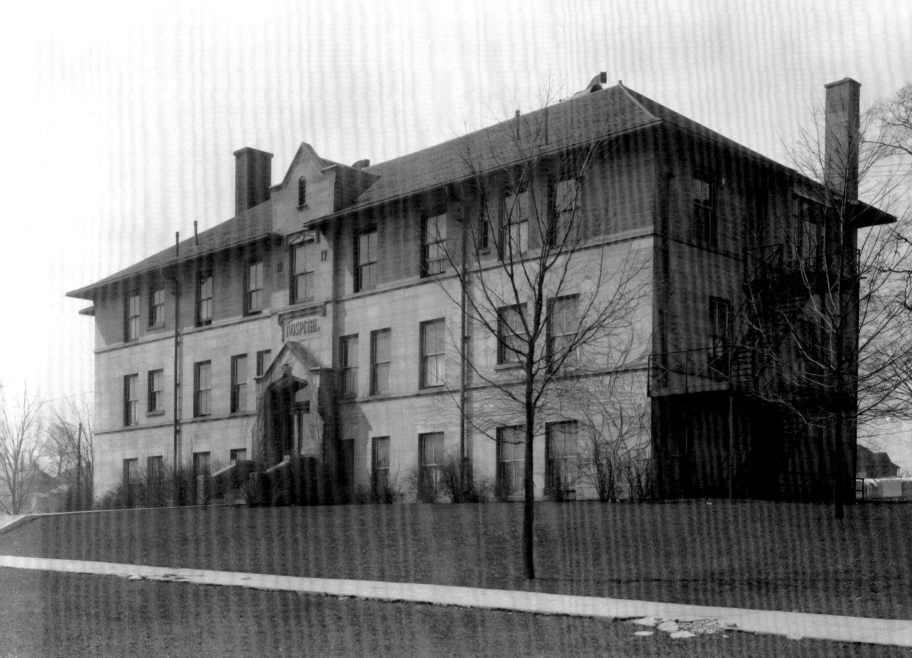

March 1918. One council member, Mrs. J. K. Beck, told of the need for an adequate building to care for the sick in the community and that a larger hospital was really a "war measure," wrote Wahl. Beck stressed that the hospital belongs to everyone in the community and all should feel the responsibility of finishing its construction.[18]

Soon thereafter, the council renewed a building campaign and the design created by the architect was used to raise money. In August 1918, it entered into a construction contract for $27,900 to cover the shell of the building, walls, basement, roof and fire escapes. The council also decided to turn the original red brick building into the nurses' living quarters.

But the Local Council of Women recognized it needed the county government's help to finance this expanded building, Wahl explained. In September 1918, the County Council of Defense promised to stand behind the council's building committee and secured Liberty bonds totaling $30,000, used as security for borrowing that money to help complete the building. A second contract for other building expenses was let for $20,000, and the council also paid for building materials from its funds. The estimated cost of the finished building was $60,000.

But funding of the new hospital hit a snag. Yet the Local Council of Women members didn't let that stop their progress.

At a meeting in June 1919, it was reported the Monroe County Council and County Commissioners had approved a $50,000 bond issue, the amount necessary to complete the hospital and retire the debt, Wahl wrote. But the bond issue had to be approved by the State Board of Tax Commissioners, and it was learned in October 1919 that body refused to allow the bonds to be sold.

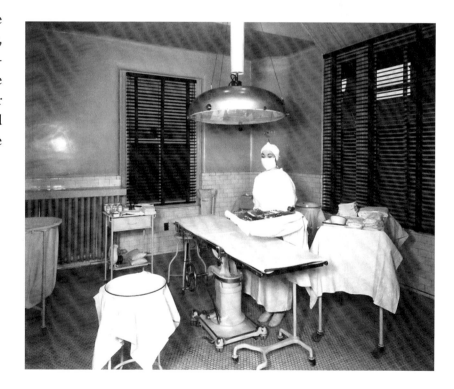

Facing, Exterior view of Bloomington Hospital's three-story stone building built in 1917. Above the door, chiseled into the limestone, is the word "Hospital" and above that on either side of the window is "1917." *Photo credit: Monroe County History Center Photo Collection, Bloomington, Indiana.*

Right, Operating room in early history of Bloomington Hospital. *Photo credit: IU Health Bloomington Hospital.*

County Judge J. B. Wilson, who supported the Local Council of Women, had drafted a bill a few years earlier that permitted the county to appropriate money for building a hospital. While the bill had passed the Indiana General Assembly, legal complications had developed over sanctioning money for this purpose, according to Wahl's report. When the State Board of Tax Commissioners refused to allow the bond issue, the governor called a special legislative session in 1920 and lawmakers passed an act removing the tax board's particular power. The County Commissioners then had full power to issue the bonds and did so, allowing the building to be completed.

"While this was a crushing blow, the women of the Local Council were undaunted and their courage and enthusiasm withstood this setback," wrote Wahl.

The law empowering the County Commissioners to issue bonds for financing the hospital also provided the body must appoint at least one-half of the 12 members of the hospital board which received money in this way. The Local Council of Women members, however, still handled the management of the facility, as well as the finances, while they also hired an administrator who was a nurse.

The Local Council of Women's hospital board appointments, Wahl stressed, were strong ones who became leaders of the board. She wrote that in the years after more men were appointed by the Monroe County Commissioners, the Local Council's female appointees often rose to the hospital board chairmanship. Wahl said she believed that was true chiefly because the women could devote the long hours required by the position and because it seemed to be an unwritten tradition.[19]

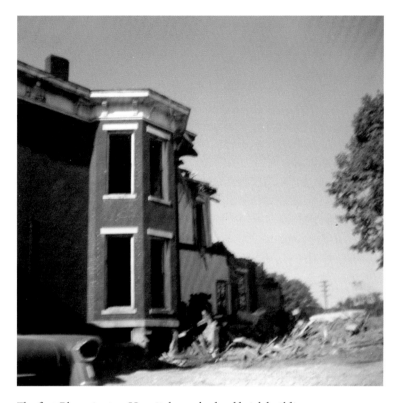

The first Bloomington Hospital, a 10-bed red brick building, with two-story bay window is being demolished to make way for the new 35-bed, three-story hospital. *Photo credit: Monroe County History Center Photo Collection, Bloomington, Indiana.*

Facing, Exterior shot of three-story stone building built from 1917 to 1919 with 35 beds. *Photo credit: Monroe County History Center Photo Collection, Bloomington, Indiana.*

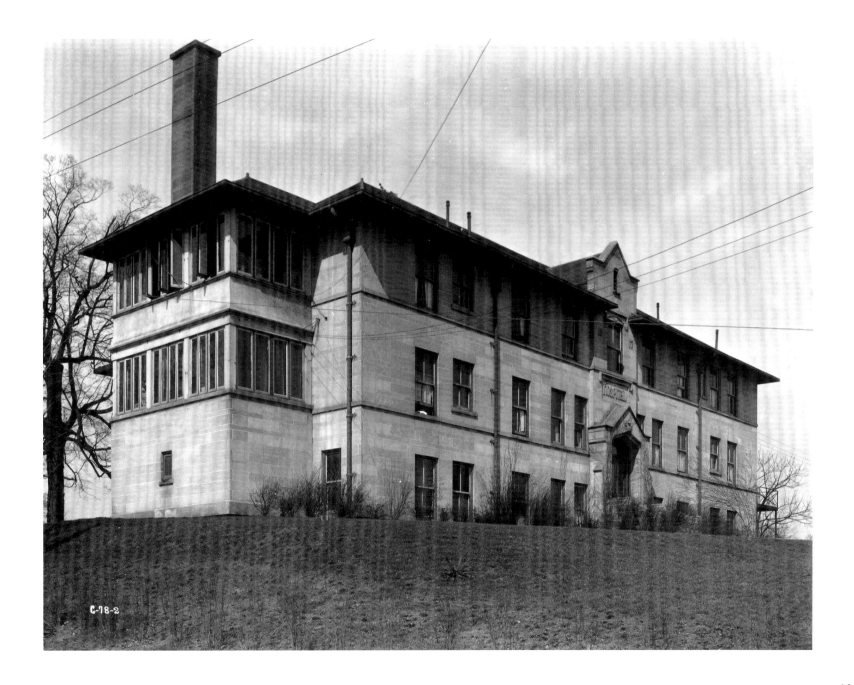

C-78-2

Frank Vilardo, former director of undergraduate programs for the IU School of Public and Environment Affairs, was the first man to serve as hospital board president, although male members served on the council for a number of years, beginning in 1960 when the County Commissioners appointed men. The Local Council of Women made its first male appointment to the hospital board in 1983.

Hospital records showed 78 patients were admitted to the new facility in 1920. At that time, patients included a large number of indigent people, unemployment was high and the country was dealing with serious diseases, such as polio, which threatened public health.

Clearly, the times were challenging, economically and healthwise.

Given the new, enlarged, three-story hospital with a 35-bed capacity, the Bloomington Hospital was able to serve the local community and several neighboring smaller towns for many years.

The Local Council of Women described its members' individual high standards and their philosophy of care guiding their operation in an October 1951 brochure. "Owned, operated and supervised by women whose home standards of cleanliness, sanitation, general housekeeping and neighborliness were of the highest type, it established a reputation for efficiency and solvency—two rare and essential qualities of any hospital," it read. "The interest of these women founders never wavered and continues through many of their descendants who are devoted to the welfare of the hospital to this day."[20]

But, again, they had to respond to the needs of the community and plan for the future.

With the population growth in Bloomington and at IU and problems arising due to returning World War II veterans, the Local Council of Women recognized in 1944 the hospital was badly in need of more beds. This time, they turned to a federal grant to help pay for a hospital expansion.

Yet some people in the community at this time questioned whether federal authorities would wish to award a grant to a hospital board comprised solely of women, according to the council's history penned by the council in 1951.

But the concerns were unfounded.

"Federal authorities replied decisively that in investigating a hospital as to its eligibility for a loan or grant, attention was given to efficiency, solvency, and service to the community, not to the make-up of the board," the historical document. "On these requirements, the rating of the Bloomington Hospital was high, and the members of the Local Council of Women stood for their traditional rights. They were magnificently upheld by the community. Harmony had been the rule from the beginning."[21]

So, the council requested and received a $92,000 federal grant in 1945 for hospital construction. Once more, the community responded generously and matched the grant dollar-for-dollar with $92,000 in donations. Still, the grant and matching funds weren't enough to develop a unified facility. A local bank, confident of the council's management of the hospital, floated a loan (amount not specified) to fill the funding gap, according to Snoddy.[22]

With all of these funds, a new wing was built directly in front of the older building, connected to it by architectural devices to create a new unified facility more than double its former capacity. The bed capacity increased to 75 beds and 25 bassinets from 35 beds in the Hopewell House.

In the council's history written in 1951, the three floors of the hospital are described in detail and illustrate the types of equipment and facilities being using and services being provided at that time. The new wing allowed some modernization and more specialized services.[23]

The new wing's first floor housed administrative and business offices and the registration area, as well as a large room with a library that was used for lectures and board meetings. Dining rooms, kitchens, service rooms and laundry facilities, all well-equipped, were also located on this floor.

One of the most modern radiological departments, according to the council's history, was located in the west wing of the first floor. This made available to residents of Bloomington and surrounding areas complete diagnostic services and X-ray treatment of cancer, tumors, and skin diseases. A "deep therapy machine," as described by the council, was primarily used to treat cancer and ailments beneath the skin and was equipped with the latest devices for directing rays to the proper areas.

An addition to the therapy room illustrated the community's support for the hospital. The walls and ceiling of the room were lined with lead, the cost of which was underwritten by the Cancer Control Society of America. The gift, arranged by the local chapter of the Cancer Control Society, is an "excellent example of community cooperation with the hospital," said the council's history.

The hospital's second floor had 50 medical, surgical, and pediatric beds. On the third floor's east wing, the maternity division was equipped with the "most modern utilities, nursery, formula room and sterilization services." The west wing housed the operating rooms, emergency surgeries, labor room, delivery room, clinical and pathological laboratories, and service utilities.[24]

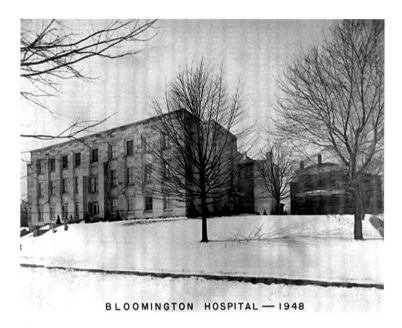

BLOOMINGTON HOSPITAL — 1948

Bloomington Hospital outside photo in 1948.
Photo credit: IU Health Bloomington Hospital.

With these improvements in the expanded hospital, the council was pleased with its success in upgrading the facility and improving services provided to a growing population in Bloomington.

"Now, the Local Council of Women of Bloomington was the sole owner of a plant worth $650,000, a plant that had grown from the humble beginnings made by a few staunch pioneers who did not hesitate to assume the responsibility of a $90,000 mortgage, despite a starting capital of only $400," wrote Snoddy.

"The ownership and operation of the hospital had germinated so gradually that few realized what a rare phenomenon in

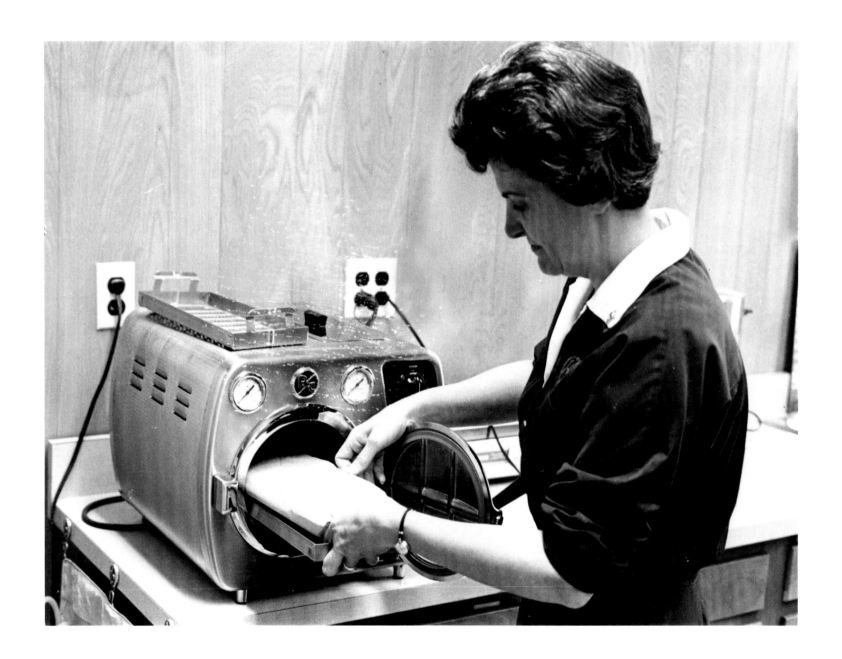

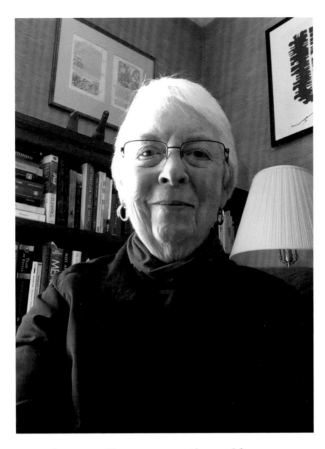

Nancy Boerner, a Bloomington resident and former IU Wells Library librarian, has been a council member since 2000 and now is serving a second term on its board. *Photo credit: Nancy Boerner.*

Facing, Bloomington Hospital nurse using medical equipment in an undated photo. She is identified only as county nurse Joanne. *Photo credit: Monroe County History Center Photo Collection, Bloomington, Indiana.*

hospital histories this was," she added. "Long practices had accustomed the women to answering the needs of the hospital, and the torch had been passed from generation to generation."[25]

The council's long-standing determination to operate and fund the hospital through the generations is one of the qualities of council members that has impressed Nancy Boerner. A Bloomington resident and former IU Wells Library librarian, Boerner has been a council member since 2000 and now is serving a second term on its board.

"They were able to sustain this for many years," she emphasized. "They must have been a fairly educated group of women." Boerner added that the council women also managed the hospital for a long time and recruited other groups of women to get behind the hospital project, too.

Boerner, who now writes the council's newsletter to its estimated 70 dues-paying members, said, "It kind of shows you what women can do, if they put their minds to it."

The second-half of the 1900s provided even more challenges and an evolving role for the Local Council of Women in operating Bloomington Hospital. These female leaders continued to adapt and to meet those challenges.

3

REACHING MILESTONES AND MAKING "OUR BEST . . . THE VERY BEST THERE IS"

LONG-TIME BLOOMINGTON industrialist Sarkes Tarzian said "the hour of decision truly is upon us," in imploring local residents to throw their financial support behind a new hospital addition.[1]

Bloomington Hospital board chairwoman Jane Wallace hoped to be able to look every patient in the eye and say, "Our best is the very best there is."

And top hospital administrator John H. Shephard predicted the planned hospital addition "will help bolster the community economic welfare and will have a direct bearing on the city's future industrial growth."

All three leaders realized the critical importance of expanding and improving hospital facilities in Bloomington in the mid-1960s. They knew the community needed and deserved better health care. They all were determined to persuade everyone they could to support their efforts to make the new hospital a reality, too.

The population of Bloomington was growing in the 1950s. Indiana University's student base was expanding. People were attracted to this picturesque small town for its natural beauty, the university atmosphere, educated residents, and flourishing business community. More doctors were beginning to move here, too.

With the generous financial help of the community and a federal grant, the Local Council of Women, a nonprofit organization that owned Bloomington Hospital, just had a new addition constructed in 1947 that brought the capacity to 75 beds and 25 bassinets.

But within a few short years, council members and the community quickly recognized the hospital had to be enlarged again to provide enough space for more beds, increased services, and modern technology to help attract top-quality physicians, nurses, and staff. By 1960, Bloomington's population exceeded 31,000.

Yet describing the brick and mortar buildings, construction, number of beds, and equipment doesn't shine a light on the dedicated people who continued pushing the hospital forward, the depth of their strong feelings about the hospital, and their commitment to offer the best health care possible to local residents.

Those sentiments were felt and expressed all the way back to the early 1900s by the original Local Council of Women members and their descendants, the Men's Advisory Council, which helped study the need for an expanded hospital, board of directors members, health care providers, and business and community leaders who wanted a first-class hospital here.

Hospital board chairwoman Wallace so eloquently put those feelings into words when she spoke to the "Three-for-One Committee" of Bloomington business, professional, and civic leaders in the early 1960s. She was making a final push to raise money to build a new 147-bed hospital, connected by passageway to the existing hospital facility built in 1947.[2]

The total campaign goal was initially $4.1 million, with a $1.3 million grant authorized under the federal Hill-Burton Hospital Survey and Construction Act, and $2.8 million from local sources. The cost increased to nearly $4.7 million when the community agreed to pay more than $650,000 to shell in two additional floors for future expansion.[3]

During the Three-for One Committee meeting, Wallace asked members if they experienced "sometimes how one little scene imprints itself on your consciousness, so that it is remembered long afterward?" According to an editorial column under her name in the *Bloomington Herald-Telephone*, Wallace then said she carries one of those scenes in her memory and wanted to describe it so they could see it, too.

"It is of a bed in a hallway, one of our rather dim and narrow hallways, I came upon it while my mind was elsewhere, and before I realized it, my gaze had met that of a boy—a rather thin, dark-haired, dark-eyed boy, not a small child," she said in the editorial. "You know—just that age when a certain masculine dignity has been learned, but when it is still necessary to remind oneself sometimes that Big Boys Don't Cry.

"He was sitting up in the bed, and as he looked at me, I seemed to see fright, and a refusal to admit to being frightened, embarrassed at being found in bed in such a place—a look which invited sympathy and yet would have been affronted had sympathy been offered," she remembered. "I knew such a young boy once, rather well, and wished I could stop and talk with him; but I dared not intrude."

With a sad recognition, she continued, "All I could do was to attempt a brief and friendly smile, and walk on, saying in my heart: 'I'm sorry, son. We're doing the best we can.'"

Wallace, though, asked, "But are we?

"As a community, are we doing the best we can when any patient has a bed in the hall or must delay his admission because of lack of space or go home sooner than his doctor would really wish if the space were not needed for another sicker person?" she asked.

Wallace praised doctors who are capable of taking advantage of every advance in medical science. But she said the people of Bloomington deserve the finest care offered to any people anywhere. "Our (board's) job now is to help everyone to see that they can have this care if they will provide the facilities for it."

She made her final plea by saying, "We would like to be able to look any patient in the eye and say, not merely that we are doing the best we can, but that our best is the very best there is."[4]

That sentiment has persisted since then.

That same sentiment has led to the hospital administration, physicians, nurses, and other health care providers advocating for and accomplishing significant milestones from mid-1900s and beyond that have improved individual and community health outcomes. Their long-standing efforts have developed and brought to Bloomington advanced medical care and technologies that people otherwise had to seek in Indianapolis or elsewhere.

Still, along the way, the community had to go through some spirited debate to reach consensus before achieving some of those milestones. That was true of the new 147-bed hospital facility that broke ground in 1963 and was dedicated on March 17, 1965—a major achievement in modernizing and expanding the hospital. The $12.5 million facility added nearly 213,000 square feet and brought the total number of beds to more than 200.[5]

One person who clearly remembers reaching that milestone was Pat Bartlett, president of the Local Council of Women at that time. Speaking to the local Argonaut Club in April 2003 about the hospital's history, she said, "A $3,000,000 bond issue was arranged by a local bank. I remember that as president of LCW, I had to sign the papers. I found that very scary. If those gutsy 1905 crew (council members) could set sail with an initial treasury of $400, we could continue the voyage with equal dedication and faith in our mission."[6]

While the need for expanding facilities was widely recognized by the late 1940s, hospital and independent groups worked long and hard before reaching a compromise solution.

The Local Council of Women and the Bloomington Hospital board of directors appointed a 27-member Men's Advisory Council, a volunteer group representing all segments of Monroe County, in 1948 to consider a larger hospital and deal with public concerns and opinions. The hospital's medical staff had first pointed out the need to plan the expansion. The Men's Advisory Council was tasked with organizing a planning committee and proposing a financial setup for the new building.[7]

"Criticisms, which had always been liberal, even back at the beginning in 1905, began to mount," reported Bea Snoddy, council and hospital historian, in a document tracing the hospital's history until 1965.[8]

During 1953–54, the Monroe County Council of Social Agencies set up a study group charged with determining the need for expanding hospital facilities, according to a six-page document written by William R. Baldwin of Bloomington, about the steps leading to the new hospital facility and the role of the newly formed Monroe Community Hospital Association. A coalition of concerned citizens, doctors, and Bloomington Jaycees members formed that association, and it was incorporated in December

1958. The group's purpose also was to determine how to add expand hospital coverage.[9]

The Council of Social Agencies and local residents contributed $3,000 for a survey of the community's hospital needs and desires conducted by James A. Hamilton Associates, wrote Snoddy. She said three plans were proposed in early 1957:

- Construct a 147-bed general hospital plant at a new site, with the present hospital plant converted to the care of chronically ill patients.
- Construct a 65-bed general hospital plan at a new site and continue operation of the current hospital, as a 75-bed general acute care unit for the time being.
- Construct additional facilities at the present site of Bloomington Hospital, providing the 65 extra beds deemed necessary by 1960 and then to expand and improve services as needed.[10]

So, lots of concerned citizens, business people, and health care officials all had the same end goal in mind—improve and expand hospital facilities. But they espoused different ideas on how to best accomplish that challenge.

Ultimately, the independent Monroe Community Hospital Association, which reportedly had more than 5,000 members, overwhelmingly concluded that a 100-bed hospital at a new site was the appropriate compromise in June 1957. The group reported at one of its meetings that land at the southeast corner of High Street and Moores Pike had been donated, wrote Baldwin.[11]

Yet, other citizens of Bloomington felt it would be a waste of money to build an entirely new hospital apart from the nucleus of hospital facilities already established off of Rogers Street, wrote Snoddy.[12]

In the meantime, hospital administrator Anna G. Nelson, who was hired by the Local Council of Women and led the hospital for 33 years, retired early in 1960, when the site problem was not settled. Some discontent had been brewing for a while, primarily among members of the Monroe Community Hospital Association, over the effectiveness of the hospital's leadership.

After conducting a search, the 12-member Bloomington Hospital board of directors, appointed Shephard, 33, from Tarpon Springs, Florida, in May 1960. He was selected by six board members elected by the Local Council of Women and six selected by the Monroe County Board of Commissioners.

His main task was to bring the board's proposed expansion to fruition by uniting all the groups to support one plan. That was indeed a daunting task for a 33-year-old newcomer to Bloomington. But the need was great. As late as 1962, the hospital had only 75 beds, just one for every 1,000 Monroe County residents, while the State Board of Health recommended four per 1,000 residents.

Efforts before and after Shephard was hired that were meant to bring together the competing groups weren't initially successful in reaching a consensus. Many public meetings were conducted to flesh out ideas and get feedback—both positive and negative. Major front-page articles appeared in the *Bloomington Herald-Telephone* explaining the weighty situation facing the community about the future of the hospital and its best location.

A front-page editorial on April 5, 1956, said this hospital debate was one of those rare instances when "an issue comes along that sweeps like a tornado across the entire community." The newspaper published results of a nonscientific poll it took showing 380 people favored a new hospital at a different location, while only eight people wanted to expand facilities at the present site. The editorial said the poll's results may have reflected that the Monroe County Board of Commissioners ignored the request of some 13,000 people for a referendum on the issue.

Yet the editorial recognized no convincing argument has been made yet to build a second hospital, rather than to adopt the less expensive option of adding space to the present hospital—the choice that the newspaper said it would support if the hospital can convince the public.[13]

In another front-page letter published on the same day, George Henley, long-time legal advisor to Bloomington Hospital, stressed reasons to support expanding the existing hospital. He reminded people the Local Council of Women insisted from its inception that there would be no political involvement in governing the hospital, which meant no tax dollars should be used and no political party could claim any voice in governance.[14]

The Local Council of Women, the hospital board, and the Men's Advisory Council worked with Shephard to appoint a planning committee of five members of the Monroe Community Hospital Association and five hospital board members.[15] While that group didn't reach a consensus, it finally led to executive committee members from the hospital and association successfully hammering out a joint plan in July 1960 to build a new hospital facility on the current site, Snoddy wrote.[16]

As part of those negotiations, the Monroe Community Hospital Association agreed to vote itself out of existence and transfer its funds to the Local Council of Women once the council

expanded and opened its membership to men, according to a *Herald-Telephone* article on February 16, 1961.[17]

"Opposing factions compromised on this solution and joined forces to conduct the biggest fund-raising campaign this community had ever known," said Bloomington Hospital's Report to the Community in 1976, which recapped the hospital's 70-year history and was published in the *Bloomington Herald-Telephone*. "Over $1,600,000 was pledged. That, along with a $1,300,000 federal Hill-Burton grant and a $1,800,000 loan, financed a modern 147-bed hospital, which was completed and ready for occupancy in March 1965."

Leaders of the fundraising drive advocated for all community members, businesses, and organizations to contribute. Tarzian, civic leader and owner of Sarkes Tarzian Inc., headed the campaign, which also used professional consultants.

"All the old gripes must disappear," he said in a September 7, 1961, article in the *Bloomington Herald-Telephone*. "This is our community hospital expansion program. It is absolutely imperative. . . . It is a must. Illness, suffering and pain won't wait for us to make up our minds.

"The hour of decision truly is upon us," he implored.[18]

The Bloomington community didn't disappoint. "Just as in the past, the community responded to the appeal generously and sufficiently, ground was broken for a new multi-million dollar hospital in 1963," wrote Snoddy.[19]

As part of the building plan, the original 10-room red brick house was razed in the summer of 1963 to clear the land for the new hospital. The house, purchased in 1905, was Bloomington's first hospital and later used as a residence for nurses. The home was built by Absalom "Ab" Ketcham, who worked as a station

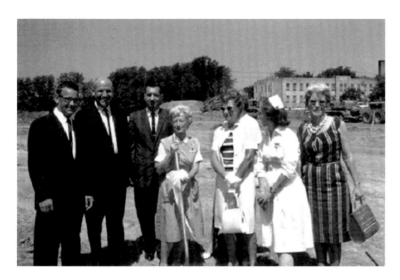

Hospital groundbreaking ceremony for the 1965 addition to the Bloomington Hospital, with hospital president John L. Shephard (far left) and other administrators and community leaders. The 147-bed, $12.5 million hospital facility, which broke ground in 1963, was dedicated in March 1965 and considered a major achievement in modernizing the hospital. *Photo credit: IU Health Bloomington Hospital.*

manager for the Monon railroad. He and his wife, Nora, sold the house to Isaac Hopewell around the turn of the century and after owning the house for less than three years, Hopewell sold it to the hospital.

While the new hospital facility was being constructed, the board of directors and the Hospital Advisory Council, a community-wide representative group, "exercised an enlightened degree of advanced planning," and decided to shell-in the fourth and fifth floors for future expansion they knew would be needed, the hospital's 1976 Report to the Community said. That move resulted in a savings of more than $1 million on the later expansion, the report added.

Converting the 1947 portion of the hospital complex into a convalescent unit never occurred because the hospital was fully occupied after only a few months, according to the report. The 1947 building was remodeled, floor by floor, and used as an acute care facility. The 1919 building was turned into office space and rooms for medical education.[20]

The positive impact of building this 1965 building can't be overstated, particularly in the opinions of the health care leaders like hospital administrator Shephard.

The hospital will mean all people who need hospital care in this area can be served, not just those needing the most urgent or emergency attention, Shephard said in an article in the *Bloomington Herald-Telephone* in 1964, when the fundraising drive was short just $150,000. Shephard said the expansion also will mean that hospital staff will have access to modern facilities and equipment.

"X-ray and laboratory departments will be enlarged and provided with the latest equipment," he said. "There will be more, larger and better equipped operating rooms, including a post-operative recovery room. Such innovations as electrically operated beds, in-the-wall oxygen and suction, patient inter-communication and adequate elevators will be available."

He also predicted the new hospital "will attract new doctors to the community, many of them highly regarded specialists in their fields. Several doctors, attracted by the proposed building program, have already started practicing in Bloomington."

Shephard said he expected the new facility would have a broader community impact, too.

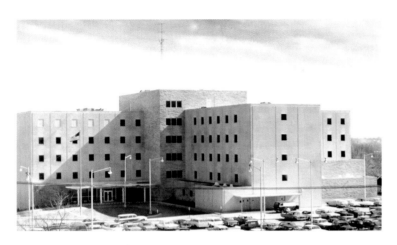

Bloomington Hospital 1965. *Photo credit: IU Health Bloomington Hospital.*

"It will also have a direct bearing on the city's future industrial growth since companies planning expansion and new plants take hospital facilities into consideration when choosing communities," he said. "And perhaps most important of all, the new hospital will stand as proof that the people of this area were concerned enough with meeting their own health needs to voluntarily pledge the funds to make it possible."[21]

Looking back, Lynn Coyne, who has had a decades-old connection with the hospital, said the expansion was pivotal to the hospital's future, and the two open floors prevented the hospital from being restrained by its facility.

"Everything else was built on the bones of that hospital. It was designed to enable that kind of growth and expansion. They (hospital leaders) had good vision," said Coyne, an attorney of counsel with Bunger and Robertson who formerly chaired the Bloomington Hospital board of directors.

"It was a bold move forward for the entire community and certainly for health care and the hospital," said Coyne, now an IU Health South Central Region board of directors member. "That was like a turning point."

MODERNIZATIONS AND MILESTONES THROUGH 2005

This updated new facility opened in 1965 was a giant step forward for the hospital and the community. The physical building continued to be upgraded in the 1970s, 1980s, and beyond.

But a wide range of other advances and improvements also occurred during the last half of the century involving the caliber and number of health care providers, hospital leadership, the types and breadth of medical services, preventive care provided inside and outside the hospital, and technology and state-of-the-art medical equipment.

Yet, many health care and community leaders stress that other less tangible factors and behind-the-scenes changes also have helped the hospital thrive and, ultimately, improve health care delivery. These changes were happening on many fronts—and several were considerably overdue, recognized some Bloomington doctors. During interviews, physicians, nurses, board members, and community leaders associated with the hospital highlighted these positive factors that improved the hospital's standing:

- Having a progressive, educated community that wants and supports good health care.
- Attracting more physicians who are specialists in different medical fields.

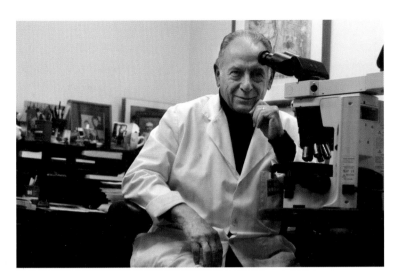

Dr. Anthony "Tony" Pizzo, a pathologist, came to Bloomington Hospital in 1951 and set up the pathology laboratory, which he directed for 49 years. Pizzo, who died in 2015 at age 93, also proposed and pushed to reality one of the first laws banning smoking in public places in Indiana. He was a member of the Bloomington City Council, which passed the ordinance in 2003. Here, Pizzo sits in his office at Bloomington Hospital on January 1, 2003, with a new microscope. *Photo credit: Jeremy Hogan,* Bloomington Herald-Telephone.

- Developing a collegial working relationship between doctors and nurses.
- Selecting new hospital board of directors and leadership.
- Changing the management of the hospital and the Local Council of Women.
- Creating a strong relationship between Bloomington Hospital and IU.
- Giving nurses more authority and training.

This significant period for the facility also is highlighted by major advancements in medical technology and its integration into Bloomington Hospital. Two key improvements in this era were an X-ray department and pathology laboratory. In January 1948, Dr. William J. Stangle set up an X-ray department with one diagnostic X-ray and a therapy unit, according to the hospital's Report to the Community in 1976. Previously, people needing X-rays had to travel to an Indianapolis hospital to get them.

In the summer of 1951, Dr. Anthony "Tony" Pizzo, a pathologist, came to Bloomington Hospital and set up the pathology laboratory, which he directed for 49 years. Hospital technicians were performing some routine lab tests before that time. But tissue specimens had to be sent to Indianapolis or Columbus or even kept for weekly visits of "circuit" pathologists from Columbus, said the Report to the Community.[22]

Dr. Larry Rink, a long-time cardiologist who arrived in Bloomington in 1974 as a specialist in internal medicine, spoke highly of the major role that Pizzo played in professionalizing the practice of medicine throughout the hospital.

"Doctors are supposed to be teaching other doctors how to do things," said Rink. "That's how we progress our profession. Some people don't continue that role of lifelong education. But Tony Pizzo was academic in how he looked at things. As a pathologist in a hospital, they get to look at all the things that are done.

"Pizzo played a huge role in doing that at a very professional level here," Rink stressed. "He was the guy—he was always interested in unusual cases and willing to take the time to do that.

"For this hospital, he was huge," Rink added.

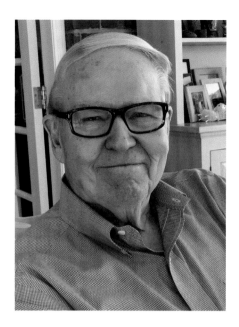

Dr. Jean A. Creek, now retired, came to Bloomington in 1955 as a general practitioner after serving as a physician in the US Army, became an internist in 1970, served as a hospital staff physician, and served as medical education director and IU professor of medicine. *Photo submitted by Dr. Jean Creek.*

Another physician, Dr. Jean A. Creek, who came back to Bloomington in 1955 as a general practitioner after serving as a physician in the US Army, also cited the impact of Pizzo on the entire hospital. Creek said Pizzo worked with the hospital board to create progressive changes at the hospital and in the community to improve health care.

Creek, now 92, who graduated from the IU School of Medicine in Indianapolis in 1949, said he also witnessed significant changes in the hospital's organization, facilities, and the practice of medicine in general, which he said were sorely needed in the late 1950s and 1960s.

When he came to Bloomington to initially work for the IU Student Health Service, Creek said, the ranks of physicians, especially specialists, in town were thin. He stressed the hospital lacked some updated facilities and services. The only doctors, Creek recalled, employed by the hospital were Pizzo and two radiologists, one of whom worked part-time elsewhere. The proposed new hospital expansion, completed in 1965, was being debated at the time.

"I can name every doctor when I came to town," recalled Creek, who also was an IU athletic physician for the men's basketball and football teams in 1955–56. "There were 47 doctors at the time, including four from Spencer, one in Smithville, and one in Ellettsville."

When he became a hospital staff physician in 1955, he said, only one room was available to treat patients with emergencies—and the elevator to get there was sometimes unreliable. "Back then, it was probably $3 if you came to the emergency room," remembered Creek, who was a general practitioner at the time before becoming an internist in 1970.

Creek said he observed that changes really started happening when the Monroe County Board of Commissioners put some "new blood" on the hospital board of directors in 1959–60 and hired Shephard as administrator in 1960. He specifically mentioned board members Wallace, wife of the dean of the IU School of Law, and Dottie Collins, assistant to IU President Herman B Wells and wife of the dean of the IU faculties, and several other members who understood the needs of modern medicine at that time.

"The commissioners picked some good women in town who got things done," he said. "They decided to put in people who would spend time on the board . . . and start to build a new hospital. That was a very significant period in 1959–60."

The time period was notable, too, because its new administrator Shephard moved to modernize the hospital's financial systems.

For the first time in the history of Bloomington Hospital, its administrator proposed an annual operating budget to the board of directors, according to a *Bloomington Herald-Telephone* article on June 28, 1961. Less than a year after he was hired, Shephard told the board and the Men's Advisory Council that his budget for fiscal year 1961–62 "represents an educated guess made after several months of study and searching for trends."

He told the two groups that an initial budget was "quite difficult to develop with accuracy" because he didn't have any basis for comparison with past years' finances, the article said. Consequently, he said he was "conservative in predicting census (patients) and income items and rather liberal in estimating expense items."

At that time, Shephard predicted an average of 61 patients per day, 1,323 annual births, 980 operations, and estimated expenditures of nearly $701,500. He called the budget essential to "provide a constant means of evaluated the administration of the hospital." The board passed his budget, and an improved financial system with monthly updates was created.[23]

The 1960s also was a decade of advances in the organization of the hospital's ongoing fundraising efforts to support its emphasis on growing facilities and improving services.

The Hospital Auxiliary, known as the "Pink Ladies," was chartered in 1961 and provided an effective base of volunteers and a source of monetary gifts, according to "History of the Local Council of Women, 1950s–1980s," written by member Cecilia

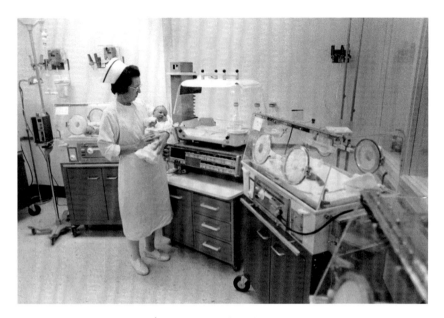

Nurse holds newborn baby (no other specific information available; photo from hospital centennial PowerPoint).
Photo credit: IU Health Bloomington Hospital.

Wahl in 1995. Volunteers performed many tasks for the hospital, including running the gift shop from which net proceeds are donated to the hospital's operating funds.[24]

The Bloomington Hospital Foundation of the Local Council of Women was established in 1965 with a treasury of $3,000, to centralize the work of fundraising, after three years of planning and research, according to the foundation's website. The work was previously undertaken by council committees. The inaugural Hospital Benefit Ball took place at the College Mall in 1966 with comedian Joan Rivers as the entertainment.

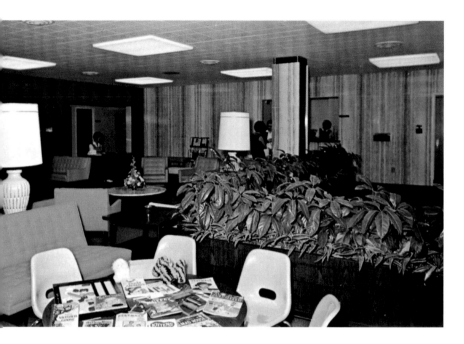

Left, Bloomington Hospital lobby, complete with plants, books and toys for children, in 1967. *Photo credit: Monroe County History Center Photo Collection, Bloomington, Indiana.*

Facing, Bloomington Hospital under construction in June 1964, building the major facility added to the hospital in 1965. *Photo credit: Monroe County History Center Photo Collection, Bloomington, Indiana.*

The foundation, which was incorporated in 1967, changed its name to the Bloomington Health Foundation in 2018. Throughout the decades, major donations were filtered through its board and financial support was provided for equipment for the intensive care unit, operating rooms and the emergency room in the 1970s, hospital expansion in the 1980s, and many other major initiatives after that period, including sponsoring the Hoosiers Outrun Cancer 5K race. [25]

New Services, New Top Administrator

Prior to the move to the new building opening 1965, the hospital administration recognized the lack of some critical services for patients and made moves to address those issues.

The hospital didn't have an in-house pharmacy, recalled Creek. "There were very few emergency drugs dispensed through Stout's Pharmacy, which was in the bottom of the eight-story building on the square. They would deliver the drugs, but there was no pharmacist there after 10 p.m. or so. If we needed some emergency drug, (we) had to get the pharmacist out of bed and get him there. The (hospital) didn't put a pharmacy in until it built the hospital wing."

In addition, the hospital set up a one-room emergency center and a pediatric unit, and services including physical therapy and respiratory therapy were being offered for the first time by the mid-1960s, said the 1976 Report to the Community. New therapists and health care providers also were hired during this period to provide these services. [26]

"Women guided the hospital's growth and development through the 1960s," said Susan Wier, former president and current member of the Local Council of Women. "They were the only board members. You could not be a member of Local Council of Women if you were an employee of the hospital. They wanted to maintain the independence and integrity of the hospital and not be overly influenced by employees to lay out a different agenda," explained Wier.

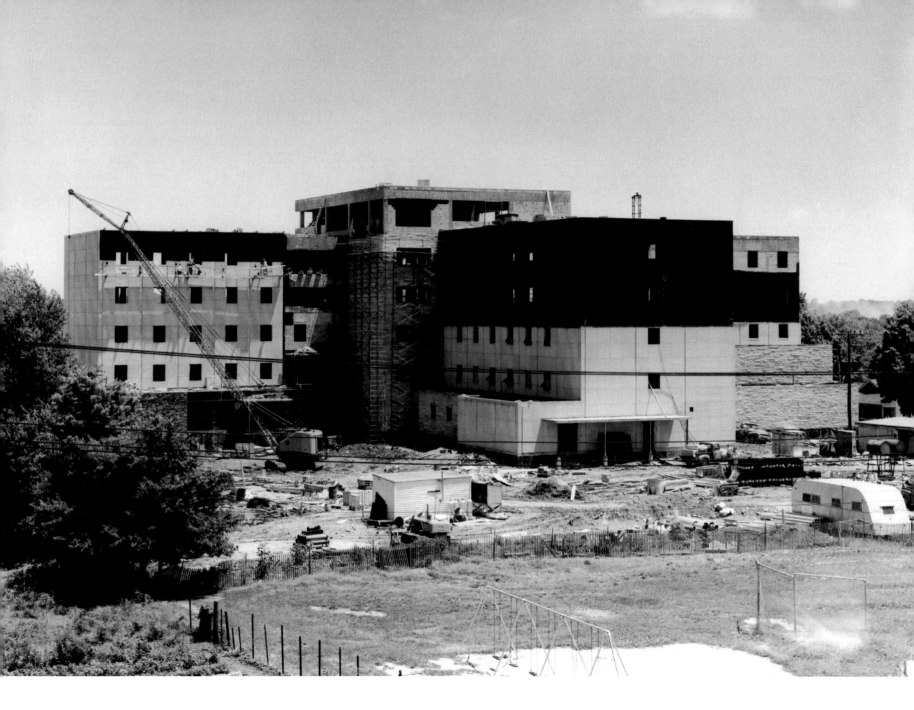

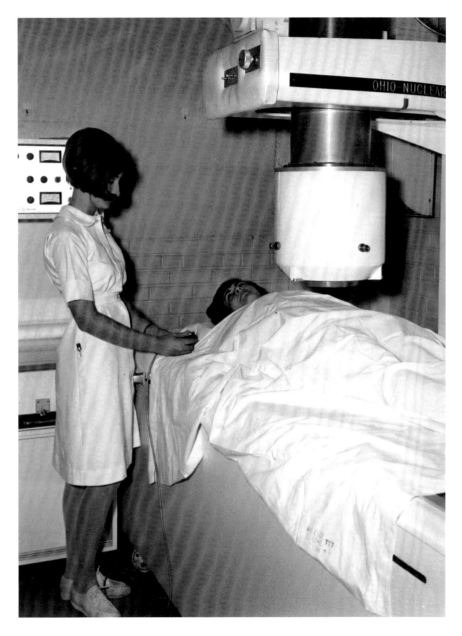

Since the beginning of the Local Council of Women, its board has served as a training ground and a conduit for membership on the hospital board, explained Wahl in the "History of the Local Council of Women, 1950s–1980s." For many years, she said, the outgoing council president was customarily appointed to membership on the hospital board for two three-year terms. The hospital board was comprised entirely of women until 1960, when the Board of County Commissioners—an appointing body along with council—first appointed men, she wrote.

Those hospital board appointments are important because the members chose the administrator. Probably the most significant personnel change in the 1960s was the hiring of Roland "Bud" Kohr as CEO and president after Shephard resigned to take a new position out-of-state in 1966. Kohr remained at the hospital's helm for 28 years until 1995 when he retired after overseeing facilities expansions, opening of the state's first dedicated cardiac care unit, and the addition of the

A Bloomington Hospital nurse attends to a patient getting some type of a scan in this undated photo. *Photo credit: Monroe County History Center Photo Collection, Bloomington, Indiana.*

Facing, Bloomington Hospital nurse at work appears to be showing a man how to work a piece of medical equipment (undated photo). The background wall displays a mural of an African-American nurse. *Photo credit: Monroe County History Center Photo Collection, Bloomington, Indiana.*

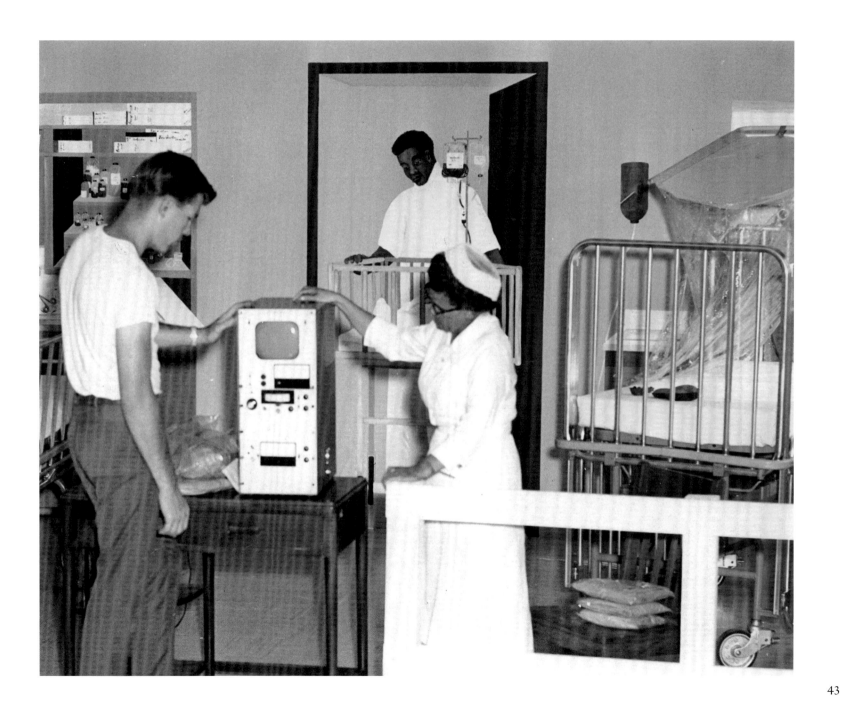

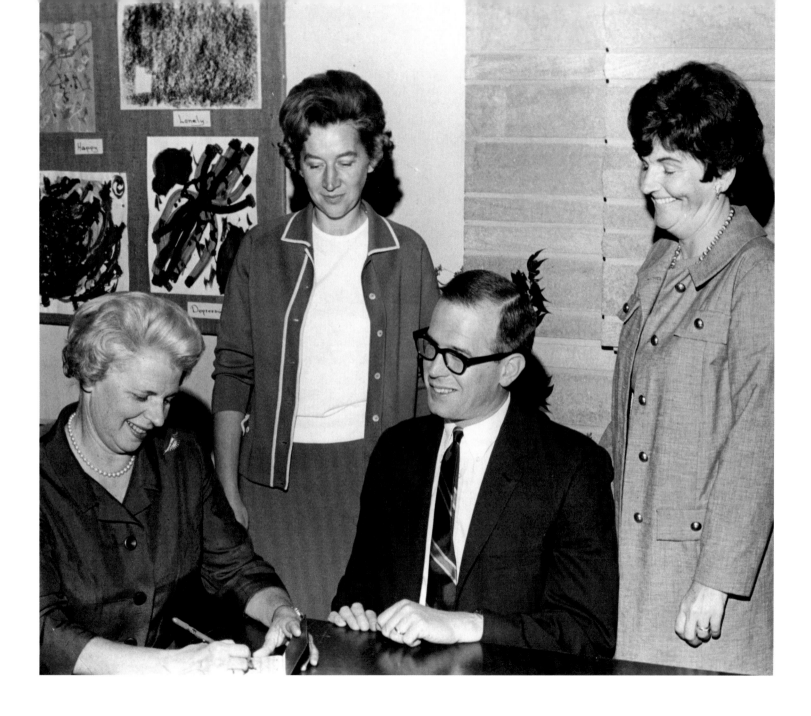

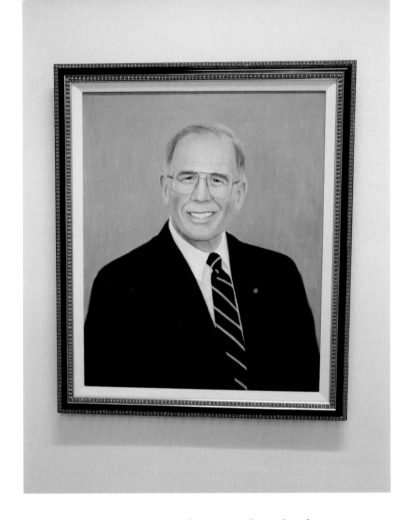

Above, Roland "Bud" Kohr served as CEO and president for 28 years from 1966 until 1995, when he retired after overseeing facilities expansions, opening of the state's first dedicated cardiac care unit, and the addition of the Outpatient Surgery Center, Radiation Oncology Center, and numerous other improvements. He died in 2015 at age 83.

Facing, Bloomington Hospital administrator Roland "Bud" Kohr meets with three women, Mrs. George Weber (standing, left), Mrs. Hogue (seated, no first name available), and another unnamed woman. *Photo credit: Monroe County History Center Photo Collection, Bloomington, Indiana.*

Outpatient Surgery Center, Radiation Oncology Center, and numerous other improvements.

"Mr. Kohr and his administrative team are credited with bringing Bloomington Hospital into a leadership position within the state of Indiana," wrote Wahl in the "History of the Local Council of Women, 1950s–1980s."[27]

But Kohr, who died in September 2015 at age 83, was just as well known and admired for the way he treated employees and all people with respect and dignity at the hospital and in the community.

For the hospital's centennial celebration in 2005, he described what he learned most about working in health care in a February 21, 2005, article in the *Bloomington Herald-Times*. "You don't really need a master's in healthcare administration, as long as you show respect to the people with whom you deal and grant them integrity," he said. "Get out of their way and don't try to tell them how, but give them objectives and let them do it themselves."[28]

Gene Perry, who worked in hospital administration with Kohr for 26 years, said that Kohr "inverted the typical organizational chart of the hospital" and put the needs of his staff before his own, in a *Bloomington Herald-Times* article the day after Kohr's death.

"I think a lot of staff at Bloomington Hospital, in the earlier years when we were a smaller organization, considered Bud to be a friend, even though he was the chief administrative officer of the hospital," said Perry, who was hospital personnel director, senior vice president, and later president of IU Health Paoli.

"He was patient. He would listen with an open mind," stressed Perry, who died in 2018. "He would deliberate, and he would make decisions, and he would be fair."[29]

The Beginning of Cardiac Intensive Care Unit

Soon after the completion of the hospital addition in March 1965, the hospital established one of the state's first cardiac intensive care units in 1967. Creek ranked the cardiac unit as one of the initial milestones that led to improving the way medicine was practiced at Bloomington Hospital. At the about the same time, Creek recalled, the hospital upgraded anesthesia practices, which allowed surgeons to do more and bigger surgeries.

Creek said he, Dr. George Poolitson, and Dr. Cyrus Houshman decided to look into the possibility of a cardiac care unit for the hospital. So they visited the Miami Heart Hospital, which was one of the first hospitals in the country with a cardiac care unit that was dedicated to treating people with serious or acute heart problems. These units specialize in the care of patients with heart attacks, unstable angina, cardiac dysrhythmia, and various other cardiac conditions that require continuous monitoring and treatment.

"We decided we could do that well in Bloomington, and our only problem with financing it," said Creek. After returning from the visit, Creek said, the three doctors talked to the head nurse operating the hospital at the time when the Local Council of Women was in charge. They asked about funding possibilities for this valuable service.

The funding quest led to asking local philanthropists John R. and Ione Figg for support, which they agreed to provide. For many years, John Figg ran his own wholesale food distributing business, which was bought in 1963 by Wetterau, a food wholesaler where he was general manager. Ione Figg, a founding member of the Bloomington Hospital Foundation, also served on the hospital board. "She was one of the members who carried over when the hospital board made a significant change in 1959–60," said Creek.

After that occurred, Creek said two thoracic surgeons came on board at the hospital. "That all made a big difference and helped upgrade the level of care at the hospital," he said.

The cardiac care unit operated in six rooms that had been designated for pediatrics on the hospital's second floor. Creek said the beds were converted to monitored beds, and the equipment's electronics generated a lot of heat, so extra air-conditioning had to be installed.

This unit led to some significant additional responsibilities given to nurses, which was a positive, liberating change in the practice of medicine, according to Creek. "If the unit was going to be right, you had to be able to shock (patients) immediately, within two or three minutes to get them back without brain damage," he said. Up until then, he explained, nurses weren't given the authority to do this or take some other steps on their own.

At this time, though, limited treatment was available for patients who had heart attacks, other than to give them nitroglycerin, explained Rink. Bypass surgery was just starting elsewhere, stents weren't being done then, no other drug treatment was available, and the catheterization lab was yet to be developed, he added.

But this was a significant first step.

Facing, Bloomington Hospital exterior view, estimated to have been taken in the 1970s, based on the cars. *Photo credit: Monroe County History Center Photo Collection, Bloomington, Indiana.*

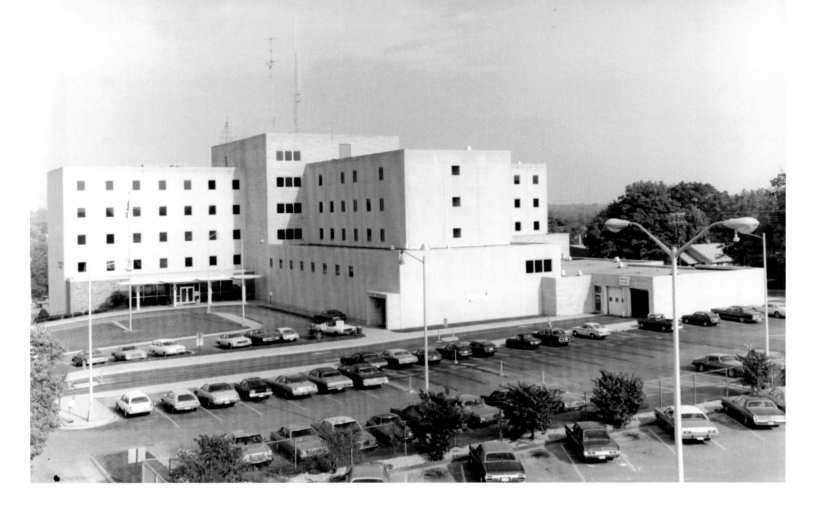

Once again, the Local Council of Women and the hospital board were faced with the need to expand the hospital due to continued population growth and greater health care needs. Less than five years after the completion of the new hospital in 1965, a fund drive headed by industrialist Tarzian and IU President Wells was conducted for another expansion.

"The area response was tremendous and over $2 million was pledged. A federal (Hill-Burton) grant of $270,000 was allowed to help defray the cost of expanding outpatient facilities and the balance needed was loaned by local banks," said the hospital's 1976 Report to the Community.

Construction of the $5.2 million expansion began in August 1970 and was completed in 1972. A total of 159 beds were added to the hospital to bring the total capacity to about 300 beds,

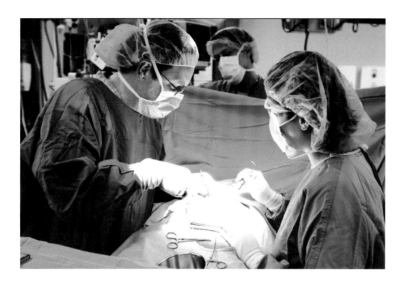

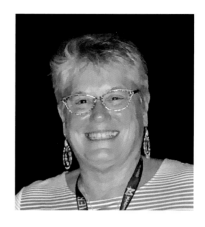

Above, Two doctors are operating on a patient (no other specific information available; photo from hospital centennial PowerPoint). *Photo credit: IU Health Bloomington Hospital.*

Right, Debra S. Wellman, who joined the hospital as a unit secretary in 1972, began her nursing career there as licensed practical nurse in 1975, starting a 45-year career as a registered nurse, educator, and nurse administrator, who is now associate chief nursing officer–practice. *Photo submitted by Debra Wellman.*

according to the hospital's Report to the Community in 1976. The total capacity included additional beds added on the fourth and fifth floors, which had been shelled-in during the original construction of the main building, the report said.

Plus, additional service spaces were built on the ground, first, and second floors, including the expansion of laboratories, X-ray, 24-hour emergency care, surgery, dietary, central sterilization, and housekeeping. The hospital also purchased new diagnostic

and ultrasound equipment in the early 1970s. An important advancement also was made in 1972 when the Medical Education Department was established, in cooperation with the IU School of Medicine.[30]

At this point, only physical therapy, medical education, volunteer services, and a portion of maintenance remained in the 1919 and 1947 buildings, according to the RATIO Architects' Historic Resource Assessment in February 2019. The portions of these buildings that were not used by Bloomington Hospital were remodeled and leased to the Community Mental Health Center as an outpatient clinic. In 1978, the Mental Health Nursing Unit was moved to the third floor of the 1947 building, known as the Kohr building, which led to its extensive remodeling.[31]

One nurse who had a front seat and was instrumental in changes in the nursing staff began her service at the hospital during the 1970s. Debra S. Wellman, who joined the hospital as a unit secretary in 1972, soon decided a career in nursing was the right calling for her. She started as a licensed practical nurse in 1975, beginning a 45-year career as a registered nurse, educator, and nurse administrator. She now serves as associate chief nursing officer–practice.

"Through my years of employment, I have completed two degrees and one certification, all the time being supported by the organization and leadership who valued professional growth and development," said Wellman.

"I have also valued our organization's commitment to values. We practice our values of team, excellence, accountability, and mutual respect (T.E.A.M.) each and every day, recognizing that it (takes) every single employee's commitment to achieve excellence in care and service." She said the hospital always has been an organization open to ideas and criticisms and responsible to changes necessary to improve patient care.

During this time period, she vividly recalled, working as a nurse in the intensive care unit that opened in 1965 with the new addition. "I remember the race track layout of our unit, with 12 beds surrounding a nurse's station that truly only visualized three of those 12 rooms. We had cardiac monitors on the five patients in the front hall and a roving cardiac monitor to use on other patients as needed. We couldn't print out any of the cardiac rhythms with these monitors, however, they did help us monitor the patient's heart activity and really improved the patient's care."

Wellman also said that during nightshift hours, the ICU team would recover patients who had surgery after the normal surgery hours. "We would take vital signs and check dressings and provide pain relief for these postoperative patients prior to their transfer to another floor," she said. While working in the ICU, she said, nurses cared for patients who had major surgical procedures, patients involved in motor vehicle accidents and trauma, and patients with respiratory and neurological diseases.

She said it was a major step when Dr. Richard Rak, a neurosurgeon, joined the hospital family. "He was very active in performing brain surgery on patients who had experienced traumatic brain injury from accidents or neurological events. The ICU was quite flexible and learned new skills and competencies as new surgeons and medical physicians arrived."

In that period, Wellman said, she learned so much about nursing and caring for people during their most challenging life experiences. "I am blessed to carry with me their lessons of love and compassion. When I close my eyes, I still can visualize and almost hear the many patients and their family members who made me a better nurse and who helped me learn to appreciate the little things in life."

The care of dedicated health care providers, as well as all of these facility upgrades, new programs, and technologies improved the services available to area residents. But another critical ingredient to providing first-class medical care—highly trained medical specialists—was largely missing.

That was beginning to change.

Going after Medical Specialists and Changing Medical Practices

Rink, a cardiologist who moved here in 1974, said he considered Bloomington one of the best possible places to provide good health care because of the overall attractiveness of the community, an educated population who wanted good health care, and because only one hospital was operating here. Yet he said the community lacked very many specialists, nor did it have a strong physicians' group. He stressed a strong hospital and a strong physicians' group are needed to work together to develop "new medicine," a term describing a shift in medical practices.

Even back then, it seemed to him, technology and surgical procedures would improve and evolve to shift the focus more to the outpatient arena and away from longer hospital stays. To make that work, Rink said, physicians and the hospital have to coordinate care. Creek, a family practice physician who became an internist, and Dr. David K. Johnloz, a gastroenterologist who

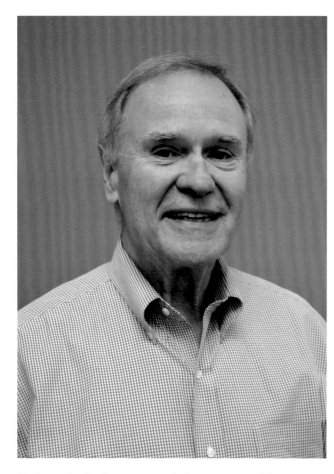

Dr. Larry Rink, a long-time cardiologist, came to Bloomington in 1974 as a specialist in internal medicine. Rink, a founder of the former Internal Medicine Associates, served as a clinical professor of medicine for the IU School of Medicine and was instrumental in starting Bloomington Hospital's cardiac rehabilitation program. *Photo submitted by Dr. Larry Rink.*

died in 1988, were practicing together starting in 1972. They then discussed forming an academic private practice with Rink, who was a full-time faculty member with the IU School of Medicine in Indianapolis at the time.

Those discussion led to the three of them formalizing Internal Medicine Associates (IMA) in 1974. Their two primary goals, explained Rink, were providing the type of high-quality care locally that patients could get at the IU Medical Center in Indianapolis and providing clinical teaching for medical students to strengthen their first two years of medical school in Bloomington. IMA was not part of the hospital, but was considered the physicians' arm for the hospital, with the exception of surgery, Rink said.

"We believed that our hospital in Bloomington needed to be able to do the most complex type of care or you would have to send patients out of the community to get care in other places— and it couldn't do that," Rink recalled.

"So, they would go to Indianapolis or the Cleveland Clinic or the Mayo Clinic. The reason I thought Bloomington could become quite sophisticated was because, one, the university was here, and, two, we had a guy named Bill Cook (owner of Cook Group) in town who was very interested in developing a large medical specialty group, and believing he could do that in Indianapolis, also. He wouldn't have to go to Indianapolis or Chicago or someplace else. IU was considered a cutting-edge university here."

Bloomington's medical services had a lot going for the community, but a major advance was needed.

"So, we had sophisticated patients. We had knowledgeable patients. We had a facility here, but the hospital obviously had to be upgraded," said Rink, 81. "But what really had to be upgraded was our medical community because we didn't have any subspecialists. We didn't have cancer doctors, kidney doctors. We didn't even have a cardiologist."

For the mid-1970s, Rink said, this situation wasn't unusual for a city of Bloomington's size. "But on the other hand, there was no reason why we shouldn't have those specialists here. The idea of all the care having to take place at the medical center, let's say, in Indianapolis for the state . . . that obviously wasn't going to last. We were going to have way too many patients and medicine was going to become too sophisticated. So, it's going to have to spread.

"My feeling was Bloomington should be the main mover of that spread outside of Indianapolis," emphasized Rink, who worked with world-wide athletic organizations and events. They included the Pan American Games, US Olympic Trials, Olympic Sports Festivals, World University Games, and the 1992 Summer Olympic Games in Barcelona, Spain, where he was US team physician.

He also said other benefits were the medical students and the IU School of Medicine, and at about this time, an idea was circulating to develop eight regional centers of health care, one of which was in Bloomington. For the next 15 years, Rink recalled, the Internal Medicine Associates virtually hired every specialist who came to Bloomington, including pulmonologists and an infectious disease specialist, except for a couple surgeons. At that time and for the next 30 years, hospitals didn't hire or directly employ doctors, Rink said, so the IMA had to figure out a way to get them to Bloomington.

"In other words, the hospital was truly a facility that employed nurses," he said. "So, virtually everything organized by the hospital was done through physicians at that time, which is different than today. If (doctors) wanted to have an intensive care unit, physicians would say this is what we need. Then the hospital would supply the facility, the doctors would set up the guidelines. The doctors would hire the doctors they needed to run that facility. The hospital would provide the facility and the nurses."

The three doctors helped direct the medical sciences program at IU Bloomington, a position Rink said they held for at least 30 years. "We were among the first in the IU School of Medicine to become clinical professors of medicine," Rink said.

Creek said Dr. Bob Robinson initially set up the medical education program with IU, and then he followed Robinson's lead. Dr. Tom Hrisomalos, an infectious disease doctor at IU Health now, followed Creek as director of medical education and professor of medicine.

"I think that combination of the hospital and the university was really important," said Creek.

When he left the medical education program, Creek said, medical students could get two years of schooling here before going to Indianapolis. "Now, all four years of medical school, students can go here now, except for pediatrics training. We maybe had 15 percent of the whole student body here. When I went to school, the first year was here, but that all changed. After that changed to Indianapolis, that's when the PhD and MD programs came here," he recalled.

"That relationship (with IU) all the way through, not any one particular year, was probably one of the most important things,

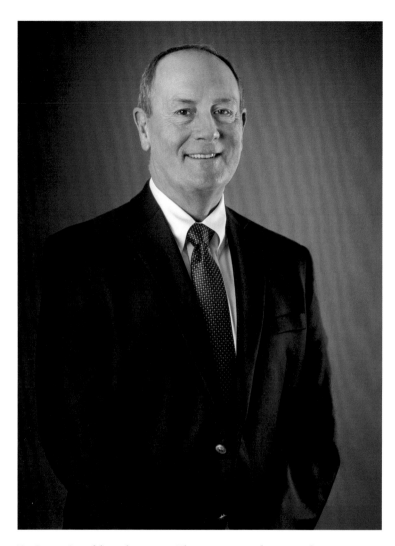

Dr. James Laughlin, a long-time Bloomington pediatrician, he is now chief practice officer of IU Health Southern Indiana Physicians. He was a founder of Southern Indiana Pediatrics, now called IU Health Riley Physicians, and the practice became part of Southern Indiana Physicians in 2011. *Photo submitted by Dr. James Laughlin.*

as far as making for better medicine and improving the hospital. Improvements in medical education affected the quality of medicine provided here," Creek stressed.

Also, current doctors were encouraged to improve their medical skills in another unique way.

Doctors in IMA, later called Premier Healthcare, took sabbatical leaves to develop clinical skills that the community needed. "We decided we would only recruit physicians who were interested in the practice of medicine and in teaching medical students, even though we were not compensated by the School of Medicine. Therefore, we were full-time volunteer faculty and taught virtually all of the nonsurgical aspects of medicine including cardiology, pulmonology, nephrology, endocrinology, gastroenterology, neurology, infectious disease, and gynecology and, of course, the basics of history and physical exam," Rink explained. Pizzo, a non-IMA member but of similar mind, was also a major contributor to the medical sciences program, Rink added.

Dr. James Laughlin, a long-time Bloomington pediatrician, has seen the relationship between doctors and the hospital change over the years from both sides. He was a founder of Southern Indiana Pediatrics, which became the largest independent pediatric practice in the state and one of the first to offer seven days per week availability and evening hours. Now called IU Health Riley Physicians, the practice became part of Southern Indiana Physicians in 2011. Now, he is the chief practice officer of IU Health Southern Indiana Physicians and serves as a pediatrician part-time.

He said Creek had the vision early on to start the IMA that attracted good physicians who drew even more specialty physicians in a wide variety of medical areas. "So they actually were the doctors who ran the hospital, in terms of the patient care. They had to be advocates for what the patients needed and what they (doctors) needed in order to take care of patients and work with the administration," he said.

Physicians always want the hospital to be responsive to their needs, he said. "But we also have to understand they (hospital administrators) have financial obligations they need to meet as well," Laughlin said. "So, when you want to provide services or get new equipment or develop a new program, it's always been a matter of who do you talk to, how do you work together. Sometimes, those things would work well, and sometimes they didn't."

Laughlin added that almost anytime he wanted something, he went to the right people, presented a business plan, negotiated with the available resources in mind, and was able to get what he needed.

However, he said it wasn't always the case that doctors and the hospital worked as a team, as they sometimes disagreed on medical or financial decisions. Speaking of decades following the 1970s, he said some physicians and hospitals formed integrated groups and became one entity.

"It allowed us and forced us to work together to provide care for the patients," he acknowledged.

Hospitals, in general, recognized they needed physicians' input and help.

"I think hospitals, as they started consolidating, realized in order for them to be successful, they were going to need a referral base that was loyal to them and would support them. So, more and more of the physicians decided to become aligned with the hospital through contracts or actually become directly employed by the hospital."

Specifically, Laughlin said his pediatric group joined Bloomington Hospital because it was better for patients and doctors. "We felt like we could have access to more services and more support and actually be the leaders of what decisions were made for pediatric care by being at the table."

Starting Cardiac Rehabilitation Outside and Inside the Hospital—Behind-the-Scenes Look

The idea that exercise and a good diet could help in preventing and treating heart disease was quite novel back in the mid-1970s, recalled Rink. "Exercise and heart disease were not two things that went together," he said.

But the idea of starting cardiac rehabilitation services for Bloomington people with heart disease started with Rink and Cook, a local billionaire entrepreneur. Cook, who died in April 2011 at age 80, was founder of the Cook Group global network of companies and a pioneer in developing life-saving minimally invasive medical device technology. He died of congestive heart failure.

At the time, Bloomington's only cardiologist, Dr. Bob Robertson, had left in 1975 and it was five years later before another one came here. In the meantime, Rink said, he and Creek handled most of the patients who needed cardiology care.

"I remember meeting (with Cook) in the Indiana Memorial Union building in 1976 and saying we needed a cardiac rehab program in Bloomington," said Rink, who was Cook's personal physician. Cook was primarily thinking of outpatient rehabilitation at a YMCA, although Bloomington did not have a Y branch at the time. Rink said he envisioned a multiple-phase cardiac rehabilitation program for prevention and treatment after heart attacks.

"We opened up a little office on 17th Street," said Rink. An IU track coach was hired to run the program, which was not affiliated with the hospital at that time. "It turned out to be exercise for people trying to prevent heart problems. It was supposed to be for people who had heart problems to come and exercise, but then we got cold feet and thought that maybe it's too dangerous for these people to exercise. But it was meant to be for community exercise and wellness, and it was also meant to be our idea for cardiac people."

Soon, they realized they needed a bigger facility.

"So, Bill thought, 'Let's build a YMCA and we'll do all that there,'" Rink remembered. The two also approached the hospital about a monitored exercise program for patients who recently had heart attacks or were having heart problems, but officials felt it was too risky and didn't want to get involved then, Rink said.

About that time, the hospital purchased nearby Hunter School, which was empty. Rink and Johnloz, another founder of Internal Medicine Associates, thought the former school would be a good site because it was close to the hospital in case a patient needed immediate medical care. In 1977, hospital officials then decided a room in the hospital could be used without charge for the cardiac rehab program, according to Rink.

"Dr. Johnloz and I literally had to paint it ourselves and did some minor carpentry work and fixed up the room," said Rink. But they needed to buy six exercise bicycles and heart monitoring equipment. "That's where Bill Cook came in. I went to Bill and said we want to have a cardiac rehab program, not just for those who are healthy and back in their lives and doing everything, but (for) people right after they've had a heart attack so they can exercise."

"Bill Cook said, 'How much money do you need'? I said $25,000. And he wrote me a check right then for $25,000," said Rink. "We were able to research and buy the best bicycles we could. There was only one other rehab program in the state, but it was in Indianapolis."

For about three years, the doctors learned as much as they could about cardiac rehab by researching the exercise results of people with heart problems or who had heart attacks. Payment from patients was divided evenly between the hospital and a fund to build a YMCA in the future because the doctors and Cook still thought most of the cardiac rehab program would end up occurring in a YMCA. The hospital realized the rehab program was working well and it wanted to be more involved, so a room in the hospital was provided, according to Rink.

"So, the cardiac rehab program grew from that," Rink said. "We got a lot of statewide and national publicity because we had a large program."

Still, Cook and Rink pursued building a YMCA, despite one consultant telling them no one would use it, while another one said it would work. "Bill and I would go out on the weekends, looking for land to buy. So, one day he called me and said, 'I just bought 17 acres, and we're going to put our Y here.'" The Southwest YMCA branch, with 50,000 square feet, was built in 1981 at 2125 S. Highland Avenue, after many fundraisers and despite major businesses and institutions not contributing funds, Rink said.

Soon, a full-time nurse was hired to run a cardiac rehab program in the hospital, and almost every physician in Bloomington volunteered to spend an hour a week monitoring patients who exercised at the YMCA program beginning in 1983. The Y's Cardiac Rehab is designed for those who have had a coronary artery bypass or heart attack or who are at risk for heart disease to help them safely regain or build their fitness level.

For more than 40 years, the cardiac program has been a huge program for the hospital, said Rink. "Now, we know cardiac programs decrease mortality and morbidity from heart disease by about 35 percent. It's as effective as bypass surgery, which decreases morbidity by 35 percent."

But he stressed cardiac rehab is not just exercise. People are taught about proper diet, and monitoring their medications, blood pressure and vital signs. "So, I'd say it's more of a lifestyle modification program done primarily through exercise. That's what we're doing today. It's changed very little today from what we were doing in 1977."

The community embraced the first cardiac rehab program and then also embraced the one at the Y, Rink said. "Cardiac rehab program is the longest continuing active cardiac rehab program in the state. I think it's probably the largest cardiac program in the state."

THE 1980S: MORE EXPANSION, RENOVATION AND HEART CATHETERIZATION LAB

One factor has been dominant during the hospital's long history: changes are inevitable. Expansion of the hospital continued to be necessary to keep pace with the population growth and medical advances.

A $24 million expansion and renovation to the hospital was completed in 1983. This addition included new facilities for orthopedics, physical therapy, occupational therapy, surgery, critical care, and a new auditorium named to honor benefactor Effie Wegmiller. The 200-seat Wegmiller Auditorium often has been used for medical education classes for physicians and medical school students and for other large meetings. The renovation added 100,000 square feet to the hospital.

The decade also was marked with the beginning of arthroscopic knee surgery, an expansion of the X-ray department, the addition of a hyperbaric oxygen chamber, and the start of the hospital-based ambulance service. In 1985, the hospital added Rebound Rehabilitation and Sports Medicine, a physical therapy facility to help people recover from loss of mobility for any reason and from sports-related injuries.

A major technological advancement, the MRI, or magnetic resonance imaging, was particularly welcomed in the community when the hospital started using it in 1988. The MRI is used to detect brain tumors, traumatic brain injury, developmental anomalies, multiple sclerosis, stroke, dementia, infection, and the causes of headache. MRI results also help doctors identify and diagnose a health issue and prescribe a treatment plan.

"How thrilling that we in the Bloomington area could benefit from this advanced diagnostic technology," said Bartlett, Local Council of Women member in a 2003 speech to the Argonaut Club. "But Bloomington has always benefited from being at the forefront of new modems of medical care because of our proximity to Indiana University. Several of our staff of highly qualified physicians teach at IU, and in the hospital the first and/or second-year medical students choose to remain on the Bloomington campus, rather than go to Indianapolis. This keeps the physicians very current with new methods of diagnosis and treatment."[32]

The decade also brought an end to the Local Council of Women's long-time ownership of the hospital properties. In 1987, council deeded the hospital properties to Bloomington Hospital

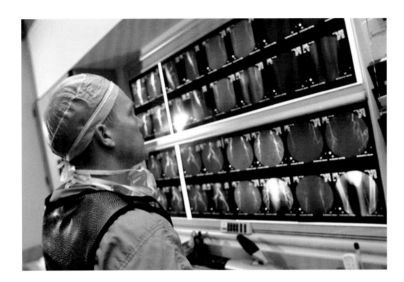

Doctor looks at series of scans (no further information available; photo from hospital centennial PowerPoint).
Photo credit: IU Health Bloomington Hospital.

Incorporated, a not-for-profit organization, according to Wahl's "History of the Local Council of Women, 1950s–1980s. The incorporation documents required the hospital had to obtain council approval to sell more than 5 percent of its assets in any given year. The council also retained the responsibility to appoint six of the 12 members to the hospital board.

While maintaining a strong presence on the hospital board, the council now also started to focus more on other health care-related projects in the late 1970s and 1980s. Members supported Meals on Wheels, the Bloomington Convalescent Center, which the council purchased and then transferred to the hospital for operations, and the Hospice of Bloomington/Greene County, which supports people in the end stage of their lives. The hospice

began in 1979 as a nonprofit organization in the community funded solely with donations.[33]

A group of concerned citizens, including Pizzo and David Smith, an IU professor of religious studies and ethics, were committed to hospice's goals. They believed Bloomington health services would be enhanced with a hospice program, so they started a grassroots effort to bring comfort to patients who were otherwise dying alone. In 1987, it became a hospital department under the leadership of Carol Ebeling and grew in staff and facilities in the following years to fill a growing need for this aid.

Developing the Catheterization Lab

Bloomington Hospital's Cook Cardiac Catheterization Laboratory opened in 1988, but the path that led to that milestone was long and not all that easy. Cardiologist Rink can attest to that, as he was deeply involved in its evolution from the beginning.

By 1980, he said, it became obvious that heart attacks were caused by blocked arteries and that people needed to get their arteries opened as fast as they could. He called it the open artery theory. Rink said Bloomington Hospital was unlikely to start a catheterization laboratory at that time, but he knew in Germany doctors had been using medicines that can be put in veins to open arteries. The treatment is called thrombolytic therapy, which dissolves dangerous clots in blood vessels, improves blood flow, and prevents damage to tissues and organs. In the late 1970s, Rink said, entrepreneur Cook, who was aware of a California doctor using this therapy, came to the hospital with a heart problem. "We gave him this drug called streptokinase," he said, adding that Cook was the first one who received the treatment here.

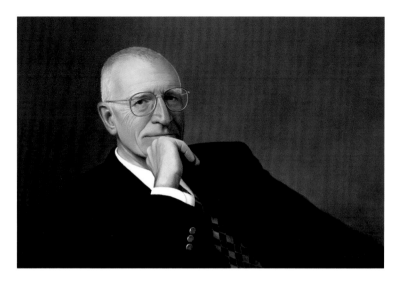

Bill Cook, founder of Cook Group, a global network of companies, and a pioneer in the development of life-saving, minimally invasive medical device technology, gave significant financial support to IU Health Bloomington Hospital and the Bloomington Hospital Foundation. Cook was major backer of the hospital's cardiac rehabilitation program and the Cook Cardiac Catheterization Laboratory. Cook, a local billionaire entrepreneur, died in April 2011 at age 80. *Photo credit:* Bloomington Herald-Times.

"So, in 1980 I started a project where everybody who came in with a heart attack, we'd give them this medicine. We did 200 patients in a row. And, it worked, amazingly. It opened arteries in a lot of people," Rink said.

"We were the first in Indiana to do that. It had been done in Germany and other places. We were learning—that's the first open artery theory. Nobody knew how to administer it or the dosages," he said. "People would come to the emergency room.

They had to have a protocol. We'd rush in and give them the medicine. . . . It was a little scary when you think about it.

"Then we decided we needed a catheterization lab here," Rink said.

The lab was opened on the second floor of the hospital, and Internal Medicine Associates hired Dr. Carter F. Henrich as a general internist and lab director. At first, the lab was a diagnosis catheterization lab, where people came when they were having chest pains: a catheter was placed in the vein and the blocked arteries could be seen, Rink explained.

"You could make a diagnosis, but couldn't do the treatment because it was believed you needed open heart surgery. Nobody in Bloomington other than me and perhaps Bud Kohr believed we could do open heart surgery. They all thought it was too difficult and those things should be done in Indianapolis," said Rink.

During this time, the IMA decided more medical specialists were needed in Bloomington. Rink said the practice started a policy of allowing doctors who wanted to get certified in a specialty to get the training and the other doctors still working would help pay their salaries during the training. "That policy allowed us to open up the cath lab. But, again, we needed money to do that. Again, we went to Bill Cook. Bill asked how much money do we need, and I told him what the hospital administration told me. He wrote me a check for that amount."

In addition to the large contribution from Bill and Gayle Cook, donations for the lab were made by employees of Cook Group, members of the Owen-Monroe County Medical Society Auxiliary and Bloomington Hospital Auxiliary, and the Bloomington Hospital Foundation's 1985 Festival of Trees and annual appeal. The lab moved to a different location in the hospital.

The next step proved harder for a different reason.

"To put in stents, we always thought you needed bypass surgery," said Rink. "But it was damned near impossible to get that done here. The medical staff voted against it and thought it was way too risky."

Rink remembered that he and Henrich then met with every physician in the community to convince them stents should be used here. Stents help keep coronary arteries open and reduce the chance of a heart attack. "We literally took the names and divided them and told them we needed this. The hospital then agreed to put the money in to buy the equipment and do open heart surgery. . . . Back then, you didn't do anything if your hospital staff didn't agree with it."

By about the mid-1990s, the catheterization lab became an interventional cath lab, said Rink. "Now, if you came to the emergency room with a heart attack, you go directly to the cath lab and we put in a catheter, blow up the balloon and open your artery."

Looking back, Rink said the hardest part was getting doctors to agree the hospital could do open heart surgery here. "But I convinced them that if we did open heart surgery here, it would be one of the five most common surgeries we would do in the hospital.

"It was, it turned out," he said. "So, it would pay for itself from a financial standpoint and the community needed it."

In 2000, *US News and World Report* listed Bloomington Hospital as a national top 100 heart hospital in the US by Solucient, a leading healthcare information provider. Now, Bloomington Hospital offers the largest open-heart surgery, angioplasty, stent placement, and cardiac catheterization program between the city of Indianapolis and Indiana's southern regions in its Regional Heart and Vascular Center.

1990S: MORE EMERGENCY SERVICES, NEW OBSTETRICS UNIT, CANCER CENTER, NEW CEO

Another decade brought another fundraising campaign to support an additional $30 million expansion and capital improvement projects affecting people who have cancer, heart problems, emergency needs, as well as new mothers and babies. Campaigns to support the nonprofit organization were necessary because it relies significantly on the public for support.[34]

The Bloomington Hospital Foundation coordinated the campaign, first considered in the spring of 1991, said foundation director Judy Talley in a January 31, 1993, article in the Bloomington *Sunday Herald-Times*. To finance the bulk of the improvements, the hospital issued $19 million in bonds. But the remaining amount had to be funded by a capital campaign that began in 1992 and hospital revenues. As part of these projects, the 1919 limestone building was demolished.

Making her case to the public, Talley stressed that not-for-profit organizations, including some hospitals, all over the country solicit funds from the public. "We've never been a county-related hospital. We've never been a church-related hospital. We've always been borne of the community," she said.

Facing, Aerial view of Bloomington Hospital taken in July 1994. *Photo credit: Monroe County History Center Photo Collection, Bloomington, Indiana.*

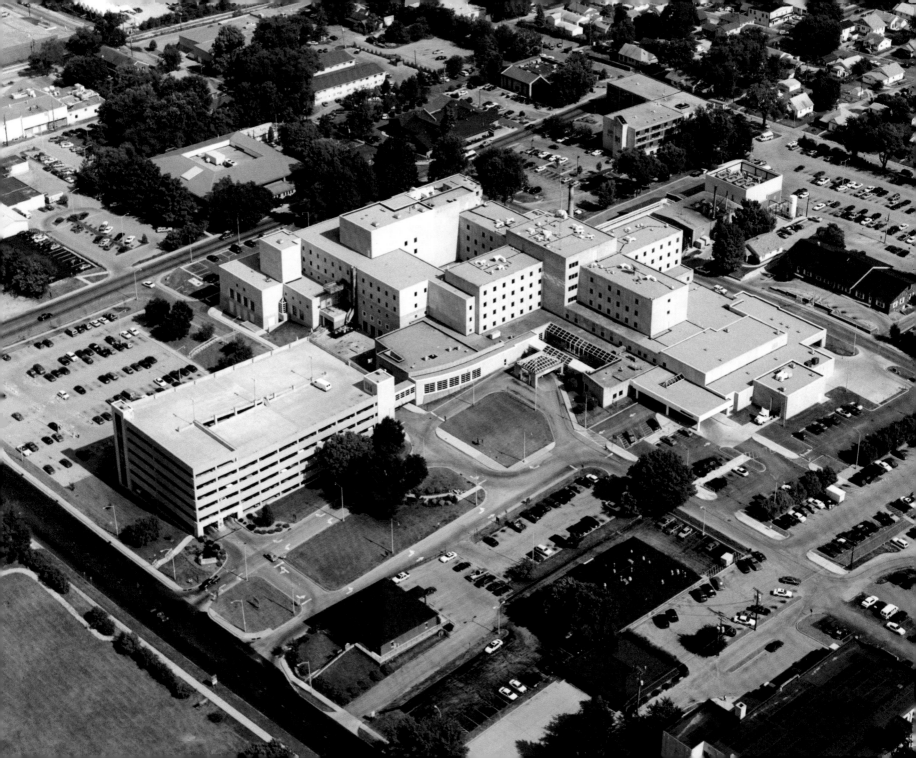

"The changes need to be made to serve the population we have," said Talley, who died in July 1997. "We didn't just decide we needed them on a whim. It was based on data. Objective data."[35]

Through this campaign, the hospital sought to provide an expanded emergency services department, a new laboratory and obstetrics unit, new facilities for cardiovascular surgery and catheterizations, an outpatient surgery center, radiation oncology center, and outpatient diagnostic center. Most of the renovations and additions were completed in late 1993 to 1995.

Kohr made a lengthy appeal for support in a long article, called "Building for Tomorrow," written as a message from him in the *Sunday Herald-Times* on December 27, 1992. He wrote: "Bloomington Hospital consistently seeks to offer and deliver high-quality, cost efficient and convenient health care services. To fulfill this commitment, Bloomington Hospital has embarked on a major expansion and renovation program."

Strategic decisions about the building program were driven, he explained, by changing medical technology, an expanding service area, and an aging population requiring more intensive medical care since they are living longer.

A total of 30 additional patient beds in the medical and surgical unit will help alleviate the hospital's bed crunch, while allowing for further increases as new physicians join the medical staff, Kohr wrote. More patient beds are needed due to increased patient volumes experienced since 1991, attributed to the recent additions of medical specialties, such as neurosurgery and peripheral vascular surgery, he said.

Kohr also made the case for a new cardiovascular program by stressing that 80 percent of area patients with heart disease still must leave Bloomington for care. He said that doesn't need to happen, as the hospital can provide a full spectrum of cardiovascular surgical services "with the same success rate as other Indiana hospitals, but at a lower cost and with much more convenience for patients and families."

The program provided 14 patient rooms, an upgrade of the current Cook Cardiac Catheterization Laboratory, one operating room with space for another, and one elevator with space for another. Kohr revealed that the hospital's first cardiovascular surgeon will be a member of the medical staff.

Kohr pointed out the emergency department's increased patient load to 60,000 people in fiscal year 1992, compared to 28,000 patients in 1983, necessitates 30 more beds than the existing 16 and a treatment system more conducive to patients. He wrote patient flow will be divided to separate low- and high-acuity patients, resulting in shortening waiting time.

The space for acute mental health services also needed to be expanded by adding seven more beds on the 5 South Wing by February 1993 and another 20 beds on the 5 West Wing by mid-1994, according to Kohr. In addition to adding new beds to the Crisis Care Center, the area also moved to the same floor as the Stress Care Center to allow for coordinating services and more efficient use of space and personnel.

Another important element was the expansion of cancer services by opening the new Cancer Care Center, now known as the IU Health Radiation Oncology Center, at Southern Indiana Medical Park in 1994. Kohr said the hospital was serving 68 percent of the general cancer population in its service area and only 55 percent of the radiation therapy population in 1992.

The goal, he said, was for the center to become more responsive to community needs, provide a full spectrum of oncology services, update treatment capabilities for adult and children, and to integrate all outpatient cancer care services.

Being more responsive to patients' expectations, needs, and safety was the motivation, Kohr explained, behind changes in obstetrics and pediatric care and additional facilities, as part of this overall expansion project. Cesarean sections and high-risk deliveries were performed in the general surgery suites located on the first floor. But the new obstetrics unit was planned to provide two surgery suites and recovery areas located right in the unit, completed in the fall of 1993. Kohr said this change would open up much needed space in the first-floor operating suites and would provide added safety for Cesarean section patients and high-risk deliveries.

Larger birthing rooms for labor, delivery, and recovery with neonatal resuscitation areas were already finished at the time of his December 1992 message in the *Herald-Telephone*. Also, the pediatrics renovation already was completed at that time. That change included downsizing of the unit in response to practices of pediatricians moving toward outpatient treatment. The renovation, Kohr explained, also increased the staff's capability to provide services to high-acuity patients who need constant monitoring in a "pediatric special care" area, relocated to the pediatrics unit.[36]

All of these changes—and many others—were experienced by Dana Watters, a long-time Bloomington Hospital nurse and administrator who started in 1979 and spent most of her tenure in obstetrics. She retired in 2015, after serving as executive director of the Regional Center for Women and Children, created in 2000.

"I had worked pretty much everything at the hospital. I liked floating and going to a lot of departments, but I always tended to gravitate back to obstetrics or ER. I enjoyed those probably the most," she said.

The earliest improvement, she said, was going from the conventional delivery room to a birthing room model, which was a national movement and started at Bloomington Hospital in the early 1980s with two rooms. All of the rooms were converted by mid-1980s. "That was, to me, a big milestone because patients didn't have to move, and patients weren't interrupted in their labor with moving from a miserable cart to another miserable cart and to a miserable delivery table. Everything was miserable about labor and delivery before then."

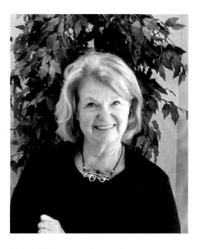

Dana Watters, a long-time Bloomington Hospital nurse and administrator, started in 1979 and spent most of her tenure in obstetrics. She retired in 2015, after serving as executive director of the Regional Center for Women and Children, created in 2000.

She said the birthing process became much better and calmer for everyone. "The births became quieter. The patient was in one room. The lights were still bright. Everything was considered sterile."

The hospital, like others around the country, reacted to women's wishes that reflected a sign of the times.

"Patients were very vocal about wanting quieter births in birthing rooms. We got that feedback from the community after women saw that in other places," Watters said. "We had to move in that direction because that is what the consumer wanted.

Women's health care was the first consumer-driven health care specialty ever. It was part of the feminist movement of the 1970s. It started a little with having who you wanted in your delivery room. It continues today. Things change in OB to meet the needs of science and the consumer."

Doing Cesarean section births in the obstetrics department rather than in a regular operating room in 1995 was also an excellent move, Watters said. At Bloomington Hospital, she added, about 20–25 percent of approximately 2,000 deliveries a year are C-sections, so it was challenging to get them to operating rooms.

"It wasn't fast," she recalled. "It was not uncommon for that to take at least 45 minutes, and I only tracked the emergencies."

But she said making that change to birthing rooms created a "huge learning curve because all the nurses had to learn how to do surgery. Everybody agreed it had to be done, but it required a lot of additional training. Nurses had to train about two years to be able to work in the operation room for C-sections. It took an additional mindset and skill set for nurses. It was tough. But now it's standard for nurses to do that."

While Watters valued the improved facilities and practices, she also said she appreciated the working environment at the hospital and the relationships between physicians and the nurses and patients. The physicians' attitude toward their patients was more of a "let's work together when I'm determining your health care, not an attitude that says I know what's best for you," she said. That relationship, she added, was different than she had experienced elsewhere.

Also, she always noticed a good collegiality between physicians and nurses. She said she never had the feeling when she was a staff nurse back as early as the 1980s that doctors thought nurses had to do what doctors say because they're the doctors.

"I can remember one time calling a doctor and saying, 'I need you now.' He came now," she recalled. "I never had a doc who I worked with who didn't come right away in any emergency. I didn't have to convince them why to come. It was always that way that they trusted my professional judgment."

Besides all the improvements to facilities and services, the mid-1990s brought a new leader to the hospital when well-respected Kohr retired after 28 years as president and CEO.

In June 1995, the hospital board hired Chicago health care administrator Nancy Carlstedt as president and CEO of Bloomington Hospital and Healthcare System, the hospital's full name at the time. She previously held the same positions at the Michael Reese Medical Center in Chicago and had worked at hospitals owned by a for-profit Humana chain in Texas and Florida.

Carlstedt came to Bloomington at an uncertain time for the hospital when debate was brewing about the nonprofit corporation becoming a for-profit facility, being sold or merging with a large medical group. Nationally, similar discussions were going on at many independent hospitals.

A month after she started, Carlstedt stressed in a July 19, 1995 article in the *Bloomington Herald-Times* that Bloomington Hospital cannot survive on its own in the increasingly competitive health-care delivery world. But she said the hospital needs to negotiate from a position of strength with entities who are coming into Bloomington's health-care market.

Within the last few years, the article said, the statewide Methodist Health Group network, St. Vincent/Community Hospitals of Indianapolis, and Mooresville-based Kendrick Memorial all bought clinics or medical practices in Bloomington. Methodist and St. Vincent already had solicited the Bloomington Hospital board of directors to join their networks.[37]

Locally, the Unity Physicians Group, a new for-profit, health care network formed by three physicians and led by Dr. Dan Grossman, also made a presentation to the hospital board about forming a partnership. The physicians' group, which incorporated in January 1966, proposed an "integrated delivery system" with one business offering a complete range of health care services from primary care to specialty care to hospitalization.[38]

While Carlstedt recognized in the article the advantages of joining large networks like Methodist and St. Vincent, she also saw a major downside. "The downside is a loss of autonomy," she said. Bloomington residents may need to travel to Indianapolis under such arrangements to obtain certain services that should be offered here, she said. But she also stressed Bloomington Hospital was not under any immediate pressure to decide and that many options were open for debate.

The deliberation continued into 1996 and also focused on the pros and cons of the hospital becoming a for-profit institutions for the first time in its 90-year history. Carlstedt didn't advocate for a shift to for-profit status, but hired a consultant to spell out the hospital's potential best options.[39]

Some local physicians, including pathologist Pizzo, opposed the hospital becoming a for-profit facility. Profits would benefit shareholders, instead of providing additional health care services for the community, Pizzo said in a January 21, 1966, article in the *Sunday Herald-Times*. He also stressed that nonprofit hospitals,

in exchange for having tax-exempt status, are legally required to provide a range of "community benefits," such as caring for the indigent, community education, and health-care services that don't produce revenue.[40]

While the hospital was owned by a nonprofit corporation called Bloomington Hospital Incorporated, it was technically owned by the now 18-member hospital board, which would have to approve any sale of its assets. But the Local Council of Women also has to approve any lease or sale that involves more than 5 percent of the hospitals assets, which were $123 million in 1994.

Although the debate was a controversial topic for several years, ultimately, a sale or merger did not occur during Carlstedt's seven-year tenure. Yet this wasn't the end of the debate, of course. But the hospital did take steps to extend its market area and increase revenue in the last years of a financially challenging decade.

In 1996, the hospital purchased from Unity Physicians two urgent care centers—Promptcare East on East Third Street and Promptcare West on West Third Street—to provide treatment of minor injuries and illnesses. In addition, the hospital took over operation of Orange County Hospital in Paoli and operated outreach clinics in other rural counties. The hospital merged with the Bloomington Convalescent Center and the Public Health Nursing Association, which added nursing home care and home health care.[41]

Before the end of the decade, Bloomington Hospital leaders realized that yet again it was time to plan another major expansion project that would create further improvements to the hospital. And hospital officials also had the fortunate task of planning the hospital's 2005 centennial celebration.

Before forging ahead with the expansion, the hospital administration surveyed staff and patients to get feedback on their priorities and changes they think were necessary to provide better services and health care. They indicated the need for more space, larger rooms and more convenient access to hospital services, according to hospital officials in a January 16, 1999, article in the *Bloomington Herald-Times*.[42]

At the turn of the 21st century in early 2000, the hospital began a three-year, $34 million expansion project to create better access to outpatient services, a cancer care unit, more outpatient surgery suites, expanded obstetrics and neonatal wards, and renovations of several other medical areas. Specifically, the project included building a two-level, 98,000-square-foot addition and renovating 82,000 square feet of existing hospital space, according to a May 23, 2001, *Herald-Times* article.

Increased demand for certain services has crowded a number of areas, including obstetrics, cardiology and radiology, and hospital admissions increased, causing patients to sometimes wait for rooms, hospital officials said. The expansion and renovation of the hospital was financed with a combination of bonds and reserve funds.

Specifically, the project

- Developed a second-floor addition on the west end of the hospital for a new obstetrics ward. It was next to the pediatric ward, which gave the hospital a unified area for maternal and child medicine.
- Created a smaller first-floor addition for new outpatient surgery registration and waiting areas, and a chapel.
- Added more parking for employees and patients and a realigned entry drive from west Second Street. The hospital's parking garage was built during the previous 1989–93 renovation project.
- Added more rooms and beds for newly admitted patients to the hospital.
- Renovated space for services, such as cardiology, radiology, neurology, endoscopy, and three outpatient surgery suites, designed around an "outpatient mall" concept.

Overall, the project is needed because the basic design and layout of the hospital dates from the 1960s, when most people who entered a hospital were likely to stay for a week or more, Carlstedt said in the *Herald-Times* article on May 23, 2001. Now, with more surgery and other services done on an outpatient basis, she added it's increasingly important to help people get in and out of the hospital in a convenient, comfortable manner.[43]

Looking back at that period, current hospital CEO Brian Shockney said an important medical milestone was the transition to more outpatient surgical interventions, leading to laparoscopic procedures, state-of-the-art robotics, and other innovative methods. These surgeries are less invasive and have shorter recovery times that often don't require hospitalization, he said.

When medical residents come out of training, they expect new equipment and services to be available, and long-time doctors need additional training to update their skills and maintain their medical licenses, explained Shockney. The hospital's role is supporting physicians with the latest technology and properly equipped surgical rooms, he added.

"We had to have a different type of surgery area and flow, where patients can come in and get their surgery and come right out," Shockney said. The physical structure of the operating rooms, the equipment, and the training of nurses all had to be updated to accommodate the changes in operating procedures many times over the years, he explained.

A different driving force behind the planning of the early 2000s hospital project was the need for more and better spaces for babies and mothers.

At the time, Watters told the *Herald-Times* in the May 23, 2001, article the expanded facility was needed due to a significant increase in the number of babies in the 1990s, which was expected to continue, as well as more hospital efforts by the hospital to serve a nine-county area, and a federal law requiring insurers to cover at least a 48-hour hospital stay for mothers and new babies.[44]

In the new wing, 17 rooms were available for labor and delivery, up from 10 in the previous unit, and a majority were equipped with hot tubs. The unit also included 22 postdelivery recovery rooms, four of them handicapped accessible, two nurseries (one for special care babies), three lactation rooms, two rooms for parents of special care infants, and a three-bed recovery and testing area for moms in need of closer observation. The special care nursery accommodated 15 infants.[45]

Looking back on the improvements, Watters said the administration recognized that not only did mothers need more beds, but space for the special care nursery also wasn't adequate. While Bloomington Hospital always had a special care nursery, the overall neonatal specialty started improving at medical centers and Riley Hospital for Children and, as a result, more babies survived who hadn't previously, Watters explained.

"We were lucky that Dr. Laughlin did his residency at Riley when a lot was going on, and then he came here and brought a lot of improvements," she remembered.

"He pushed, shoved and made us be where we needed to be with special care for newborns. So, it was exciting at the time to see babies do better," Watters said. "It started with survival, then it went to survival and less lung problems. Now, we've gone to survival, and less lung problems for their whole life."

She said the neonatal intensive care unit (NICU) progressed to improve babies' physical developmental care by putting them in the right positions, compared to being in the womb, and improving the environment to keep down noise and eliminate bright lights.

The bigger neonatal intensive care unit that opened in January 2002 was a significant development, she said, because of better facilities. But Watters also said the nursing staff improved, educational opportunities increased, and the hospital recruited good physicians and then a neonatologist, who is a pediatrician with additional training in neonatal care.

"To be in NICU, that's been one of the most exciting things in my career," Watters said. By the time she left, the neonatal unit had a neonatologist and neonatologist nurse practitioners.

"That was a huge milestone for Bloomington," she stressed.

Financially, though, the early 2000s were challenging years for the hospital.

Costs were rising and operating revenue was decreasing for a number of reasons, Carlstedt said in a *Herald-Times* article on October 9, 2001. She instructed department heads to reduce total work hours by 5 percent "without compromising care" by reducing overtime pay, hiring fewer temporary workers, and reducing full-time hours to 37.5 hours weekly.

The fiscal year ending in September 30, 2001, had operating income after expenses of $1.72 million, compared to $6.97 million two years earlier, and payment reductions in government Medicare and Medicaid programs and private managed-care plans have kept income from growing, reported Carlstedt and chief financial officer Jim Myers in the article. In addition, write-off for bad debts and charity care in 2000 totaled about $13 million, the highest figure ever, they said.[46]

But in November 2001, the hospital board members announced Carlstedt's contract that ended in June 2002 was not going to be renewed because they wanted to "explore new avenues of leadership."[47]

The following May 2002, the board selected Mark Moore, 49, chief operating officer of Community Hospitals of Indianapolis, as Bloomington Hospital's new president and chief executive officer as of July 1. Moore, who had a 25-year career in health care industry, led the not-for-profit Community Hospitals system of four hospitals, three nursing homes and five surgery centers for nine years.

"My initial goal is to get all the hospital's different constituencies working together as we move toward consolidating our strategic plan, building on the hospital's strengths while looking at the possibility of new programs and outreach efforts,"

said Moore, in a May 25 article in the *Herald-Times*. At the time, Moore took over a 260-bed hospital with 1,925 full-time staff, 320 physicians, 17,155 annual admissions, and an annual net operating revenue of $179 million, according to hospital statistics.[48]

Amid the leadership change and renovations, the hospital experienced additional accomplishments as the day-to-day work of the staff and leadership continued unabated. According to the hospital's News and Notes newsletter's 2002 Year in Review, among the highlights were

- The Regional Center for Women and Children sets a hospital record 205 deliveries in one month in May 2002.
- The Bloomington Hospital Foundation raises more than $1 million in fiscal year 2002.
- The Olcott Center for Breast Health expands its reach to people with all types of cancer and changes its name to the Olcott Center for Cancer Education in October 2002.
- The Diabetes Care Center wins an American Diabetes Association Education Recognition Certification.
- Bloomington Hospital's Operation Heartbeat wins an American Heart Association award.[49]

The major celebration of the decade came in 2005 when the hospital recognized its centennial anniversary of the year that the Local Council of Women, a collaboration of women's clubs, came together to fund and operate that 10-room red brick house on the south Rogers site.

Moore, reflecting on the hospital's many achievements in late 2004, said in an interview that the centennial is a "celebration of a long heritage of service" and a chance to showcase the hospital's impact. "The hospital has a strong history of providing quality service, and that service is attributed to the volunteers, employees, and nurses and physicians working to serve one purpose," he said for a hospital publication.

In his second year as CEO, Moore said he wants to focus on enriching the quality of care given to patients by providing a positive environment for employees. "It's important to instill pride in our caregivers, because of who they are and what they do. They must have a sense of mission and purpose."

He stressed that teamwork between the medical staff leadership, board, and management is an essential part of maintaining a successful hospital. That strong relationship between departments provides an inviting work setting for all employees, Moore said. He added he has significantly reduced the employee turnover rate and waiting lists exist for key hospital staff positions.

Moore pointed out the hospital is in the process of applying for "Magnet status in nursing excellence," which is awarded by a national accreditation body to designate hospitals that stand out in terms of employment opportunities for nurses. (The hospital first received that status in 2010.) Not many hospitals in the country have achieved that status, he said.

Since he became CEO, Moore said, he guided the completion of a strategic plan with 28 goals that emphasized the hospital's commitment to serve south central Indiana. "We want to exceed the expectations of those we serve through technology, innovation, and partnerships," said the article called "A Large Celebration for a Large Contribution," written by Emily Walsh.

Moore also stressed that it's important to maintain a strong relationship with the community not only by providing quality

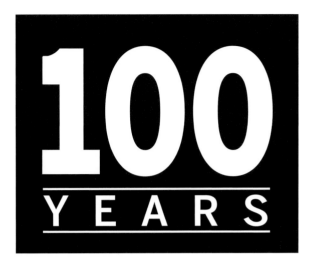

100-year hospital logo. *Photo credit: IU Health Bloomington Hospital.*

care but also by educating citizens on important health issues. "We have a lot of sophistication, like the town itself, but we're in an urban area that's small enough for us to maintain an interpersonal connection with a lot of people," he said.[50]

Kicking off the celebration, the hospital hosted a February gathering that drew 400 people and concluded with a gala event attracting more than 500 people in December. The gala, where guests were served filet mignon and bid on silent auction items, raised more than $85,000 for the hospital's financially strapped emergency services. Earlier in June, the American Heart Association also hosted a Bloomington Heart Gala, sponsored by Internal Medicine Associates and Cook Incorporated, with proceeds going to the hospital, too.[51]

During the midst of the centennial anniversary, though, Bloomington Hospital officials were looking over their shoulders.

The new Monroe Hospital at the corner of Fullerton Pike and Indiana Route 37 was starting to take shape. The $35.5 million facility, with 91,000 square feet and 28 private rooms, began accepting patients in October 2006.

Moore recognized there's "no question" Monroe Hospital will draw some patients away from Bloomington Hospital. "That will make it more challenging for us to remain financially healthy while continuing our mission of helping the ambulance service and providing indigent care," he said in a *Herald-Times* article on December 23, 2005. He added he expected significant increases in the cost of medical equipment, pension plans, utilities, and medical care for employees in 2006. To compensate for the increasing costs, Moore said, the hospital has to raise its rates in 2006 by 9 percent for the second straight year.[52]

Pressures from many sides were closing in on Bloomington Hospital to integrate with a larger health care system. Higher costs for equipment, personnel, utilities, emergency services, and medical care. More competition for patients. Less reimbursements for government health care programs. Higher costs for indigent care. And larger hospital groups dangling offers to merge.

The perfect storm was emerging.

IU Health Care Economist Says Government and Economic Influences Impacted Hospital's Growth and Future Path

Strong, dedicated community and health care leaders have guided the development of Bloomington Hospital through many challenges over its 116 years of existence.

But Kosali Simon, a nationally known IU health economist, said many government and economic influences have helped shape the city's independent hospital and led to its integration with the IU Health system. They include federal policies supporting hospital growth, major government health care spending raises, population increases, cost pressures, and mounting trends toward hospital consolidation, she said.

While hospitals in some other areas have faltered or closed, the IU Health Bloomington Hospital has survived and is now evolving as part of the Regional Academic Health Center, which opened in 2021 on Indiana Route 45/46 bypass.

"Bloomington has been fortunate to be a pretty thriving community, so it has gotten over those kinds of concerns and still maintained the hospital," said Simon, an IU associate vice provost for health science and the Herman B Wells Endowed Professor at the O'Neill School of Public and Environment Affairs. "We've had the big employers, like IU and Cook Group to help maintain employment, even when some big employers left."[53]

Simon has spent the past few years researching the impact of health insurance reform on health care and labor market outcomes, and the causes and consequences of the opioid crisis. She also serves as an adjunct professor in the Kelley School of Business' economics department, an affiliated faculty in the Data Science program, and an affiliated scientist at the Regenstrief Institute, where she is fostering health services research at IU Bloomington. She previously served on the Local Council of Women, the nonprofit organization which created the hospital.[54]

Simon, who has a doctorate in economics from the University of Maryland, College Park, answered questions about national influences on the hospital and other factors affecting its development since it first opened in 1905.

Q: What was a primary early factor influencing hospital construction and growth in the first few decades of the 1900s?

A: Some key federal policies affected the growth of hospitals, in terms of building and also financing of hospital care, said Simon. The Hill-Burton Act was significant in funding lots of hospitals, including the 1947 expansion of Bloomington Hospital, she explained.

"A lot of hospitals you see standing today were built in that time period, so it makes sense that a lot of hospitals today are now needing to decide whether they will relocate or renovate in

some way. It's not like hospitals in the US were all built at a totally random time. Any hospital you see is equally likely to have been built in the 1930s, 1940s and 1950s. There was a wave of building at that time," she said.

The Hill-Burton Act gave hospitals, nursing homes, and other health facilities grants and loans for construction and modernization. Under the community service provision, facilities using these funds must provide emergency treatment and treat all persons residing in its service area, regardless of race, color, national origin, creed, or Medicare or Medicaid status, according to the federal Health Resources and Services Administration's website. The program stopped providing funds in 1997, but about 140 health care facilities nationwide are still obligated to provide free or reduced-cost care, the website said.[55]

Q: What were significant national laws that expanded health care spending for US citizens and, as a result, affected hospital finances and growth?

A: Congress's passage of Medicare for senior citizens and Medicaid for low-income people was an important national step taken in 1965, said Simon.

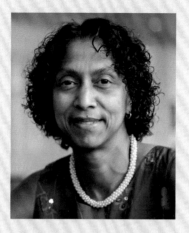

Kosali Simon, a nationally known IU health economist, is an IU associate vice provost for health science and the Herman B Wells Endowed Professor at the O'Neill School of Public and Environmental Affairs. *Photo submitted by Kosali Simon.*

"That got to have had an impact on hospital finances because it meant there was now a payer and people didn't have to just pay by themselves," she said. "Hospitals knew there would be this guaranteed payer through Medicare. Medicare now has become such a larger funder of hospital services. It's not just directly through Medicare. There are all sorts of financing mechanisms within Medicare. Hospitals get financed in lots of interesting ways."

Before these payment mechanisms, Simon said, hospitals were providing some care to people who wouldn't pay. But she said hospitals had to subsidize some of that health care, and some people didn't get the care they needed.

She also pointed out that hospital care provided in the US is very different than access to prescription medications. People can't typically get medications from pharmacies and not pay for prescriptions, Simon said. "That's far less commonly done than if you go to an emergency room and there's no possibility of payment. The emergency room doesn't turn you away. There's an expectation you will be provided life-saving care."

A well-known 1986 federal law, called the Emergency Medical Treatment and Labor Act, said Simon, mandated that people have to receive stabilizing medical care, regardless of their insurance status or ability to pay. But since its enactment, it has remained an unfunded mandate.

Q: *How did expectations for the level of care provided by hospitals change in the 1900s?*

A: "Until the 1920s to 40s, hospitals were thought of as a place where there wasn't much to do for you medically," Simon said. "You went there and you're risk of infection was higher, and hospitals didn't really know what to do with you."

But she said the ways hospitals care for patients developed at the same time as medicine developed. "Hospitals were just a workshop of the trained professionals. If the training and the knowledge wasn't there, the hospitals weren't going to be able to do anything for people at the time. So, the complexity of cases changed, along with the fact there was actual healing, rather than hospitals being just a place for taking care of the sick."

Then, health care spending really started growing in the mid-1960s, partly due to the availability of Medicare funding, she said. "Also, some people say the existence of Medicare accelerated medical discoveries because when researchers know a funding source exists, they are much more likely to undertake the discovery process, knowing that it will be expensive once the knowledge is developed. Knowing that there is a payer there makes a big difference."

Q: *What is causing hospitals to become smaller and what are the results of that trend?*

A: "The initial history is one of hospitals growing in importance, in size and in what they can do, as modern medicine advanced and knowing more types of surgeries could be done and more types of babies could be saved," she said. "The most recent phenomena is that hospitals are having to become smaller. The new hospital has a smaller footprint than the old hospitals, in terms of number of beds."

Hospitals are supposed to plan for the future, and the population is aging and growing, she pointed out. But hospitals are growing smaller because of cost pressures. "We get to a point in the medical discovery curve that we learned to do so many things, but they've become so expensive because they involve more complex work."

As a result, Simon said, the health care community is starting to move some of its services outside of the hospital. "So you have surgeries that get moved off-site to make the hospital be the place where you have the most complicated surgeries. You've got shortened stays for many types of procedures and surgeries. Yet, we're still battling ever-increasing health care costs, despite these measures that have happened."

Q: *Are shorter stays a positive change for patients?*

A: "With hospital care, people are concerned if the reimbursement system leads to financial incentives to discharge people early," she said. "In response to those kinds of concerns, the hospital readmission penalty was introduced in the federal Affordable Care Act. Accountable care organizational models are in effect now that determine how Medicare will reimburse hospitals."

People are now worrying that not enough incentives exist for hospitals to help manage people's care after they are discharged. "Some people think, though, if a payment system would pay hospitals for each time a patient gets readmitted, then hospitals would have as much of an incentive when discharging patients to make sure their care is well taken care of in the outpatient setting, such as a skilled nursing facility, or making sure they get to the next doctor's visit. Those are lots of things hospitals are doing now."

Q: *What factors have specifically affected the growth trajectory and operational changes of IU Health Bloomington Hospital?*

A: As Bloomington's population grew, the hospital grew, but some communities are declining in population, and as a result, a whole swath of rural hospitals has closed, Simon explained. A community's growth or decline largely depends on the type of industry located there, she added.

"If communities have an academic foothold in their areas, they did pretty well, especially if the flagship university was located there," she said. "But if communities relied on some types of manufacturing and those jobs were lost, the area hospitals had to figure out some way of staying open. Some rural hospitals had to close."

Another national trend among hospitals and physicians' groups is ownership changes, similar to those that occurred in Bloomington, according to Simon. Since its creation in 1905, Bloomington Hospital was owned first by the Local Council of Women, an independent, nonprofit organization, and then Bloomington Hospital Incorporated until integrating with IU Health in 2010.

"The practice of medicine has become more of a business operation that is done by large companies, rather than a sole entity run by an individual or independent hospitals grown from their own roots," said Simon.

"When faced with cost pressures and a bad financial picture, small hospitals are often approached by a hospital system that stresses its management practices and expertise and promises of saving the hospital," she said. "This has led to hospital purchases and consolidations. This was not a special phenomenon here but part of a nationwide trend."

Similarly, she said, physicians are much more likely now to practice in groups, rather than independently. These changes partly have been due to the complexity of the billing environment and reimbursements for care, she added. "There is so much complexity. It's not like the plain fee for service there used to be."

Q: *Describe the changing roles of hospitals and physicians related to making improvements in health care and to managing hospitals.*

A: "Earlier, physicians viewed themselves as independent and the hospitals were their workshops," she said. "They thought, 'We'll figure out our self-governance since the hospital exists for use to practice our art and expertise.'"

But now she stressed a growing movement exists toward hospitalists—physicians employed by hospitals. Health care still relies on physicians, but hospitals tend to hire more physicians who are not necessarily skilled in business or human relations but doctors who've had long practices, Simon explained. A similar parallel exists in academia, she said, as provosts and department chairs are all teachers, rather than management brought in without teaching experience. Now, some physicians and nurses are full-time managers, and more hospitalists are hired full-time by hospitals to treat patients, as opposed to community physicians with admitting privileges, she said.

Some hospitals are leading the way in advancing certain types of medical care, such as the Mayo Clinic and Riley Hospital for Children at IU Health, which does research on children with sleep apnea, Simon said. "So there are lots of these trials happening where they are trying to innovate and do research."

Hospitals also have a big role, she added, in addressing not just the public health concerns within their hospitals, but in their communities, too. "That's one of the things they are required to do because they are nonprofit entities. By being so, they don't have to pay property taxes or other taxes and they can raise funds through municipal bonds. They have lots of advantages, and in return, they are supposed to provide community benefits," she said. Among these activities could be community flu clinics and workshops for people to learn about managing diabetes.

She explained the value of teaching hospitals, where research is conducted on medicines, but she added a lot of research on medicines is conducted outside of hospitals. Simon also mentioned a current movement exists of physicians opening up their own specialty hospitals. "Physicians want to create their own surgical hospital because they want to run things entirely their way," she said.

Q: *What are the advantages and disadvantages of larger health care systems?*

A: "Earlier, people would talk about a hospital. Now, one talks about a health care system. That's because they are all now under the same ownership. Physicians' offices and hospitals are often are within a hospital system," she said. So, this can facilitate better transfer of information, electronic health records, and other advantages that make it appear to be a seamless hand-off of information and good communication, Simon explained.

But with that type of ownership structure, she said, all decision-making is happening at a higher level. IU Health knows about all the prescribing of physicians in community settings and what their patients are like, Simon added.

People in health care view these changes differently, she said. Physicians from earlier generations sometimes will talk favorably about how medicine used to be practiced, Simon pointed out. "But now it's the business of medicine. There are so many rules governing medicine that the autonomy is reduced," she said some doctors say. "On the other hand, we're already spending a whole lot for health care, and people find it difficult to afford. We're doing things differently in order to keep health care costs down. So it makes sense to change. I don't think you're going to get consensus from people."

Q: How do you think the new Regional Academic Health Center will evolve in the future?

A: It's very exciting to see how having a closer link to the Indiana University will progress, Simon said. While there is no plan currently underway, she said, she'd like to hear thoughts about the possibility of this center becoming a research and teaching hospital within 20 years. Whenever a stronger connection exists between a university and a hospital, she said, one wonders whether the hospital can become a training and research facility. "Certainly the fact that IU and the hospital are co-located and all of the changes that come about from that, means there is room for that relationship to grow in the future," she said.

4

DECADES OF CHALLENGES: DECADES OF SUCCESS

WHEN THE NATION'S most severe pandemic in a century struck in early 2020, IU Health Bloomington Hospital and its health care providers jumped into action—safeguarding the facility, altering operations, finding protective gear, and, most importantly, protecting and saving patients' lives.

The challenge was formidable.

But people in south central Indiana count on the hospital to take excellent care of anyone needing its medical services and expertise and to shield all patients and staff members from unnecessary health risks. Hospital leaders say that is their responsibility in the unprecedented health crisis caused by COVID-19.

Yet providing top-quality care, skilled services, and compassion is exactly what Bloomington Hospital health care providers do every day in many ways, big and small, in the hospital and community.

Their impact is far-reaching and wide-ranging.

Sometimes, their work happens behind-the-scenes, not well known in the community. Besides tending to patients' medical needs, health care providers educate the public about smart health practices. They provide social services to patients. They help fight diseases and poor health conditions in the community. They reach out to at-risk populations. They comfort people in hospice care.

And they continually work to improve the overall community health and wellness.

On a broader scale, the reputation and quality of Bloomington Hospital over the years have boosted the city's economic development efforts. The hospital's good name has enhanced the city's ability to attract top businesses and citizens looking for first-rate health care. The hospital's repute has helped attract highly qualified doctors, nurses, and other professionals, agreed business and community leaders interviewed for this book.

"The constant drive to deliver the very best care is what distinguishes this hospital and what benefits this community and the economy," said Lynn Coyne, attorney and long-time community leader and member of the IU Health South Central Region board of directors.

RESPONSE TO COVID-19 PANDEMIC

The hospital's skilled handling of the COVID-19 outbreak beginning in early 2020 clearly shows the significance of health care leaders and providers who can marshal the resources and dedication needed to meet an unparalleled challenge and take decisive actions. The hospital treated 139 people with COVID-19 as inpatients through July 15, 2020, according to Brian Shockney, president and CEO of IU Health South Central Region. As the pandemic continued throughout the year, more patients were treated, after this book's editorial deadline.

"We had to close down the hospital to all visitors at first, and then limit the number of visitors and only allow those 18 and over," said Shockney. "We went down to three entrances for everyone in the facility. We had to close down the cafeteria to anyone but our employees. We practiced social distancing within

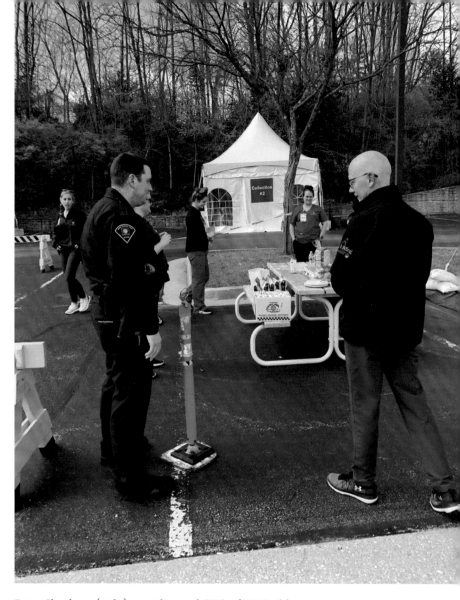

Brian Shockney (right), president and CEO of IU Health South Central Region and IU Health Bloomington Hospital, visits the hospital's COVID-19 laboratory drive-thru testing site on Sunday, March 29, 2020, and brings the team lunch. *Photo submitted by IU Health Bloomington Hospital.*

our own teams—only allowing a certain number of people in our lounge and cafeteria and even break rooms."

Keeping all employees safe was of utmost importance.

"We had to be sure everyone had masks and PPE (personal protective equipment)," he said. "Our supplier for normal supplies of drugs and PPE ran out pretty quickly. IU Health has relationships in China, one in particular that carried our brands, so we were able to secure PPE to protect our patients and staff members," said Shockney, when interviewed in late May of 2020.

"When other organizations were struggling to have enough, we had what we needed and had enough to ensure our staff and patients were protected," he explained.

Dr. Dan Handel, vice president and chief of staff of IU Health Bloomington Hospital since April 2018, said being part of the large IU Health system, with greater financial reserves, also had other benefits for the hospital and illustrates a major positive reason for integrating with IU Health in 2010.

The state put elective surgeries on hold for about a month in the spring of 2020, so some doctors, nurses and other medical staff weren't doing surgeries. But the hospital was able to continue paying them if they were willing to help out at other system hospitals when needed, he explained. The system's hospitals also were asked to shift medical personnel if necessary, and several IU Health Bloomington Hospital nurses served at different locations for a short period. Handel said the IU Health system distributed drugs, such as remdesivir, to sites in the amount of dosages required when needed.

Rooms for COVID-19 patients needed to be altered, too.

"We also had to convert two other nursing units to negative pressure rooms, with negative pressure fan units in the windows

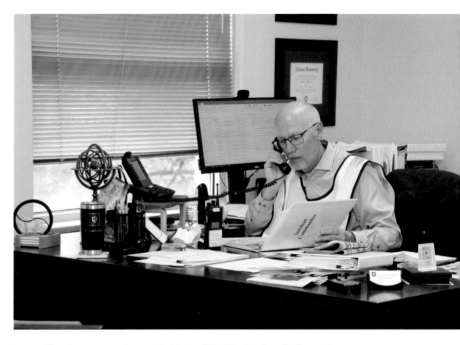

Brian Shockney, president and CEO of IU Health South Central Region and IU Health Bloomington Hospital, talks on the phone during COVID-19 incident command operation in July 2020. *Photo submitted by IU Health Bloomington Hospital.*

that pulled air through the room and blew it out," Shockney said. "We had to buy all that equipment."

But changes in facilities and equipment weren't the only crucial actions required.

"We had to practice in a very different way," Shockney said. "We had to put a lot of technology in place. Loved ones would sit in their cars and employees would take iPads to the cars. Employees would have the iPad connection and families could see the care going on and connect with the doctors at that time."

Difficult choices had to be made, quickly.

"We had to decide how to handle our patients who were passing at that time, including COVID patients and non-COVID patients," he said. "The Ethics and Values Committee was very busy during that time. They had to consider potential harm of others getting COVID from patients who were dying. Loved ones were dying of cancer, but their spouses couldn't be with them."

Shockney said the hospital had to determine when to make exceptions, such as allowing family members to go in separate doors and then equipping them with full gear. The hospital, for example, allowed one parent in a room with a child patient, but the adult had to wear protective gear and couldn't leave the room.

"We had several heart-wrenching cases—loved ones having to say good-bye to parents," he said. "We had to make tough decisions."

Oftentimes, he said, decisions were made on a case-by-case basis so different circumstances could be considered. The Ethics and Values Committee, consisting of administrators, including Shockney, nurses, behavioral health specialists, psychiatrists, and pastors, made these types of choices. They weighed the risks and benefits of certain types of contact and considered that asymptomatic people can spread COVID-19, Shockney added.

"Sometimes decisions had to be made during the middle of the night," he said. "We had to be on call. We had lots of new scenarios that had never come forward before and it takes a few of us to get our heads together and think it through. We had to figure out what's the best way to treat them (patients) and provide safety for other people and staff."

Determining the best supportive therapy for COVID-19 patients and dealing with the disease's uncertain trajectory have been perplexing problems for the medical staff, said Handel.

"I've worked in hospitals in the past that were in the path of hurricanes," he said. "We're not sure when this is going to pass, though. The lack of certainty of the timeline of this is the most anxiety provoking. It's literally a novel virus, and we are learning information as quickly as the data is coming in."

But he was proud of how well staff members performed, despite worrying about their own risk of virus infection. "I think everyone did a phenomenal job and people were willing to step up and help out at any time."

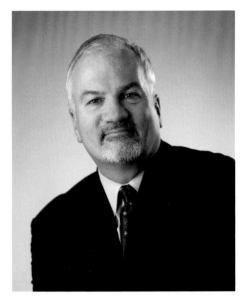

Dan Peterson, current chairman of the IU Health South Central Region board of directors, is vice president of industry and government affairs for Cook Group. *Photo submitted by Dan Peterson.*

The hospital's well-organized reaction to COVID-19 impressed Dan Peterson, chairman of the IU Health South Central Region board of directors and vice president of industry and government affairs for Cook Group. He also said this type of response is expected throughout the IU Health system.

"There is a very well-developed incident response set of plans and protocols," Peterson said. "It actually goes back to not just in this region, but it's typical across the IU Health system, and I would hope it is more common than less common."

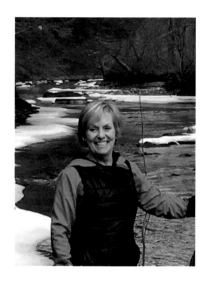

Carol Weiss-Kennedy has been director of community health at IU Health Bloomington Hospital since 2007. *Photo submitted by Carol Weiss-Kennedy.*

The protocols actually were created after the September 11, 2001, terrorist attacks, he explained. "They really helped drive making sure that when an unnatural event like this happens, that it is very clear how the teams pull together and respond to that. So there is value and effectiveness in preventing the spread and treatment of the disease, and there is power in really well-defined protocols and integration and communication across the system, both in the system and across the system as a whole."

The hospital's reaction to COVID-19, though, is broader than the treatment of patients by health care providers. It indicates one of the many ways the hospital's services benefit the whole community, as well as its collaboration with other local organizations and agencies.

Carol Weiss-Kennedy, director of community health at IU Health Bloomington Hospital since 2007, said registered nurses and licensed practical nurses in her department work with the Monroe County Health Department to do contact tracing to find people who were in contact with individuals with infectious diseases. Beginning in early 2020, IU Health nurses tracked down contacts of people with COVID-19.

"It's just amazing the partnership between the (county) health department and the hospital and how that continues to work, even in a pandemic," Weiss-Kennedy said. "It's probably even more valuable in the type of pandemic we're having."

Nurses contact people by phone and sometimes in the community directly, especially if they need to find someone in the homeless community, so they will then work with shelters, she explained. "It's very unique. There aren't a lot of programs or collaborations like that. It's a very hands-on thing they have to do," Weiss-Kennedy said.

If someone tests positively for COVID, that information is given to community health staff members. They contact that person and find out when symptoms started. They ask the person who he or she has been in contact with and activities in the last few days, and then contact people who may have been infected and ask them to shelter in place, she said.

"You can put any communicable disease in that plan—measles, mumps or meningitis—and now we have the COVID virus. So, it's a plan that public health put into place a long time ago," Weiss-Kennedy said. "It also helps guide information given to the community so not everyone is giving their version of the information."

TOP-QUALITY HOSPITAL KEY TO BOOST ECONOMIC DEVELOPMENT AND ATTRACT EMPLOYEES

The hospital's overall impact, though, doesn't only affect patients it treats or people who receive services, many agree.

"As a community, when we have companies come in, there are two things they are interesting in—schools and health care," said community leader Joyce Poling, who has seen the impact of the

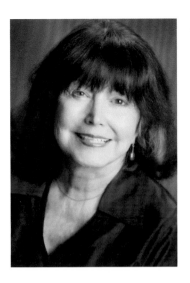

Joyce Poling, community leader and currently assistant to the chancellor for community engagement at Ivy Tech Community College's Cook Center for Entrepreneurship, was a member of the Monroe County Board of Commissioners, leader of the Local Council of Women, and a member and past president of the Bloomington Hospital board of directors when it integrated with IU Health. *Photo submitted by Joyce Poling.*

hospital in several roles. She was member of the Monroe County Board of Commissioners for 12 years during the period 1988 to 2008, leader of the Local Council of Women, and a member and past president of the Bloomington Hospital board of directors when it integrated with IU Health.

When she was a Realtor for RE/MAX Realty, Poling also heard directly from people who were considering moving here. "People coming here want to know what kind of health care services you have and what your hospital is like. People ask if the community is more generally able to provide good health care for them. Those are the kind of questions they ask," she said.

"The hospital was a plus for us," said Poling, assistant to the chancellor for community engagement at Ivy Tech Community College's Cook Center for Entrepreneurship since 2009.

She said people believe the hospital to be a top-notch facility for numerous reasons, including its neonatal unit, certification as a stroke center, accreditation as a Magnet hospital, which recognizes hospitals for quality outcomes, nurses' impact and influence, and educational accomplishments, and its good reputation.

"It is considered a good part of our vital community," Poling said.

Community leader Coyne also has had a front row seat for assessing the impact the hospital has made on people and on the city's economic development. He explained the community and major employers have played a role in the hospital's advancements due to their high expectations for health care. He's also been directly involved in the hospital's leadership over the years and was an employee decades ago before becoming an attorney.

Coyne, now an attorney of counsel with Bunger and Robertson, likes to say he was the first hospital orderly and the last chairman of the Bloomington Hospital board of directors before the hospital integrated with IU Health. Perhaps his five-year tenure as president of the Bloomington Economic Development Corporation, ending in 2019, gave him the best vantage point to evaluate the hospital's broader role.

"The quality of health care in a community is a major factor for an employer. This has many facets to it," Coyne explained.

"The largest employer (in Bloomington) is Indiana University. So you have in your community a large educational institution with highly educated individuals, who, as a result, are well-informed and have high expectations as to their health care, what's going on nationally and what's available locally," he added. "So, what's going on nationally are cutting-edge innovations that are sort of their expectations for their local health care system. That drives innovation and advancement. That drove building a new hospital back in 1965, too."

To remain in good stead in the public's eye, a city has to provide good health care and good hospital care compared to the standards at that time or better than those standards, according to Coyne. Also, he said an important factor is whether the community is willing to work toward and commit to the hospital's growth with their money and time.

Many IU employees understand the need for good health care and how medicine is advancing, and other major employers, such as General Electric and Thomson Consumer Electronics, over the years also wanted to be in an environment where their employees have good health care, Coyne said. Plus, the hospital's long relationship with the IU School of Medicine has helped the hospital maintain quality and attract top people, he said.

"The overall environment is one of a community that understands the value of good health care, and the hospital is a huge factor in that," Coyne explained. "As the hospital management desires to keep up with developments and advances in medicine, it needs to grow the facility and acquire more modern equipment and reach out to the community for financial resources.

"All of this is integrated and part of the dynamic that drives the hospital's success," he said.

As a hospital board member, Coyne said another contributing factor was the constant objective to stay current with the latest trends and developments in medicine. "Those efforts were supported by the business community. You could reach out and communicate. The hospital had the kind of leadership that wanted to move forward and continue to have the greatest quality of care. That meant bringing another doctor in and a specialist, or equipment, or both, quite often."

Peterson, a 30-year leader at Cook Group, agrees that having a strong, integrated health care system with high-quality care is a "definite, definite selling point for attraction of business and certainly retention of business, especially when you're talking about organizations that need to retain high-quality talent."

"We've had a good success in having high-quality physicians and clinical care across the different disciplines of medicine," he added. "Those are all very important. It's always IU, IU Health and Cook that are the top three employers organizationally, so they're not only attractive, of course, but they're a big part of the economy."

But he recognized that years ago, the hospital's reputation wasn't as strong.

"It's a necessity to have high quality. I would also say, and it's been a number of decades now, when things weren't as rosy at Bloomington, way back before the merger. There were times when the quality of the hospital, not necessarily the docs in the community, was under some suspect," he said, speaking of the 1980s. Peterson said former IU Health Bloomington President Mark Moore was brought in to "really turn that tide" and this hasn't been an issue since then.

For local business owner Jefferson Shreve, the importance of excellent health care in a community to drive economic development can't be overstated. "If you look at the world through an economic development lens, access to quality health care is, I'm hesitant to use the word amenity . . . but it's one of those important factors that you have to provide in a community to attract people with the options to vote with their feet as to where they are going to bring their talents and apply their craft," said Shreve, who served on the Bloomington Hospital board of directors from 2005 to 2011, as the Local Council of Women's representative.

"You've got to have it. In bigger markets, it's like having an airport with good connections and top flights that we talk about in bigger communities," explained Shreve, owner of Storage Express, headquartered in Bloomington.

While all communities want to have access to quality health care, not all of them can because it's really expensive, according to him. "You need a concentration of resources in both really smart, highly trained people, and high-cost equipment. That means that not every community can have the same high-quality access to health care. It's what differentiates a Bloomington from (other cities)—it's one of those things."

Shreve also has seen the importance of good hospital care on a personal level. He lost his father to brain cancer in 2001. Shreve said his father received excellent care at a hospital in Indianapolis, the city where Shreve was born and raised.

"When you have someone close to you that's struggling with cancer, and you see the quality of care and the services and how important it is, that hit me at a relatively early stage of life," he said.

He couldn't be involved in the health care system where his father was treated, but he wanted to find an avenue to do so here, now that Bloomington was his home and he graduated from IU. Initially, he served on the Bloomington Hospital Foundation board from 2001 to 2005 before becoming a hospital board member. He was a member when the board voted to integrate with Clarian, later renamed IU Health.

Over the years, Shreve has recognized the link between the local population and the hospital's quality.

"It's been a symbiotic development of a quality health care system in conjunction with the development of a healthy community that a lot of people choose to live in," he said. "This is a desirable place to live. People choose to live here, in part, because the community has figured out how to provide a quality health care system that's close to home. You have a quality system because you attract human talent and a lot of those professionals want to make their home here."

Put in dollars and cents, Bloomington Hospital's impact in the community totals nearly $48.8 million in many different types of community investments, according to the 2018 Community Benefits Report produced by the hospital.

Of that amount, more than $34 million was deemed for community benefit. The major contributions were $16.8 million for unreimbursable Medicaid patient costs; $7.6 million for subsidized health services; $5.5 million for financial assistance; $3.1 million for community health improvement services; nearly $500,000 for health professions education; and $444,400 for community benefit operations.

In addition, the report showed the hospital invested nearly $9.2 million in Medicare patient costs, $5.5 million to cover bad debts, and $50,250 for community building activities.[1]

COMMUNITY HEALTH PROGRAMS IMPROVE
LIVES AND HEALTHY BEHAVIORS

That quality health system encompasses programs and departments of the hospital that sometimes don't get a lot of public attention, despite the positive impact they have on individuals' lives and on groups of people with health conditions, diseases, or common health needs.

To Peterson, the community health services the hospital provides are invaluable.

"They are a really, really impactful resource and a well-designed set of programs that the (hospital) performs across the community," said Peterson.

A strong example he cited is the Nurse-Family Partnership program, which works with pediatric physicians to help address infant mortality.

The program's efforts focus on improving maternal and infant health outcomes, increasing safe sleep practices, improving access to prenatal care, and supporting mothers early when they are establishing healthy habits, according to the hospital's 2018 Community Benefits Report. The free and voluntary program supports low-income mothers with their first baby, from early pregnancy through their child's second birthday. The Indiana State Department of Health helps fund the program, and clients are also referred by Women, Infants and Children (WIC), pregnancy centers, the State Department of Child Services, and the judicial system.

Results show that the Nurse-Family Partnership program, which pairs first-time mothers with registered nurses, has had a positive impact on new mothers, according to the report.

In 2018, the program's staff served 95 clients, completed 965 home visits and saw 34 healthy babies born. Of the 33 percent of enrolled clients who smoked, 69 percent ceased smoking prior to delivery; 98 percent of clients initiated breast-feeding; 97 percent of babies were born at a healthy weight (5.5 pounds or greater), and 90 percent of babies were born full-term (at least 37 weeks).[2]

From Peterson's viewpoint, the community public health activities are critically important, especially because Indiana historically has not invested enough money into public health resources.

"We haven't put a lot of money into that, as a state," he said. "Part of what you see as a result, not just solely because of that, but we're near the bottom of every health ranking nationally. That's lifestyle, too, but (health outcomes) can be impacted by public health funding."

The nurses, health educators, and social workers of the Community Health Department, have provided a wide variety of services and programs to the public since its formation in 1997, according to Weiss-Kennedy. Its main office, called the Community Health Building, is located at 333 E. Miller Drive, off of south Walnut Street. But the department also offers programs at Hunter School, 727 W. Second Street, and at churches, schools, and other community sites throughout the south central region. The hospital annually provides more than $600,000, and grants supply about $5 million to the department, said Weiss-Kennedy.

"It's probably the best thing I've done in my life," she said, noting the positive effects of the department's efforts.

She praised the department's social workers and health educators working with individuals throughout the community who need help coping with diabetes, obesity, tobacco cessation, Alzheimer's, HIV/AIDS, nutrition, and other health concerns. She said about 70 staff members also provide support for family members and work well with doctors, who often connect their patients with the department's services.

When the department started, Weiss-Kennedy said, it was offshoot of the marketing department intended to increase community engagement. Initially, a lot of the work started with two groups—senior citizens, by helping them stay active and engaged, and students in Monroe County Community School Corporation.

Weiss-Kennedy noted one licensed practical nurse health educator, Sheila Evans, who has since died, did a tremendous amount of work in the schools. "She did tobacco education, sexual health education, substance use prevention, and a variety of things. She probably looked like she worked for the schools more than anywhere else," she said.

"That was her calling—working with schools. Her goal was the prevention of at-risk behaviors," Weiss-Kennedy recalled.

Starting in the late 1990s, Evans forged a strong partnership in schools that continues to this day, Weiss-Kennedy said. Evans had a passion for normalizing the discussion about sexual health, and Weiss-Kennedy said she did an "amazing job" talking with students in grades 5, 8, and 11. "We're still able to do that, and we're training the MCCSC teachers, so that discussion can happen any time.

"We started with health fairs within the schools and then searched for grant money to do extra programming in the schools. We created after-school programs and really tried to help students at risk," she said. "The department just grew from there."

Weiss-Kennedy said the hospital's outreach program was likely one of the first started in a city of Bloomington's size. The department soon developed community needs assessments to guide its work toward the greatest needs of the community. Every three years, she added, the department conducts surveys and holds focus groups to find out the most critical needs, based on the community's input.

IU School of Public Health and the IU Survey and Research Department helped develop a 2,000-person random sample poll mailed to homes so people can use the hard copies or fill them out online.

"We also go to different sites in community and ask to host an in-person focus group, and people just give their thoughts about what they see every day. That gets to a different population," said Weiss-Kennedy, who previously worked in occupation health for the hospital and as a Monroe County YMCA program director running the cardio pulmonary rehabilitation program.

A unique arrangement that sets Monroe County apart from other areas is the department's contract with the Monroe County Health Department, according to Weiss-Kennedy. Since 1960, the county health department has contracted with Bloomington Hospital to take care of the clinical side of the health department's duties. That means the hospital's Community Health Department does immunizations and communicable disease investigations and contact tracings, such as those for COVID-19.

"If someone has a communicable disease, our nurses are contacting them to have them isolated and find out who they've come in contact with, so (nurses) can provide education and prevention and stop the spread of the disease," said Weiss-Kennedy. Nurses have done that for tuberculosis, measles and mumps, too.

The department is the sponsoring agency for WIC, the federal program that aims to safeguard the health of low-income women, infants, and children up to age 5 by providing nutritious foods to supplement diets, information on healthy eating, and referrals to health care.

As part of WIC program, the department's nutritionists provide qualifying families with vouchers for food staples, check children's weights and heights, help them learn to prepare meals and purchase the right types of food, said Weiss-Kennedy.

Staff members provide diabetes education, nutrition therapy for eating disorders, heart disease, and obesity, information on car seat safety and bicycle helmets, Alzheimer's resource services, an infant mortality prevention program, one-on-one counseling, and clinical and social services for people with HIV/AIDS though the Positive Link program.

Weiss-Kennedy said her department has been spreading more programs, including Positive Link, to the other 10 counties, outside of Monroe County, in the IU Health South Central Region. "The new Regional Academic Health Center will give us more ability to reach out across that region. We're going to continue to serve the community and partner with organizations in the other counties."

HIV/AIDS Positive Link Program Makes a Difference

Since 1994, one of the Community Health Department's biggest programs has been Positive Link, said Weiss-Kennedy.

In the past, she said, HIV really was a death sentence. The department received grants from the Indiana Department of Health, she added, but some people felt like it was just providing funding for funerals. Weiss-Kennedy also remembered families dropped off family members with HIV at the hospital's front door and then drove away.

Bloomington Hospital accepted and brought in people with HIV and helped them during that transition period leading to death, she explained. Staff members have told her most of their time was sadly spent planning patients' funerals.

"Now, people are surviving with a higher quality of health in their lives," said Weiss-Kennedy. "That was pretty amazing. Many of the people with HIV didn't have insurance."

The Positive Link program provides comprehensive prevention and holistic social services for people with HIV, including education and testing, as well as direct services and clinical care.

This program stood out to Shockney soon after he came here in 2017 as the hospital's chief operating officer.

He learned that the program sponsors a one-mile walk on the B-Line in the spring to raise money for its activities and for buying Christmas gifts for patients. "My wife and I participated in the walk and were able to witness the amazing work of the (hospital's) care and social services team, along with the appreciation of the community that receives these services, and we were overwhelmed with pride.

"It just really moved us regarding the impact and what they were doing," Shockney said. "I realized the impact of this is big, and we can truly stop the spread of AIDS and the virus. We went to work with the team, and Carol (Weiss-Kennedy), and started to expand it."

When he began his tenure as president in 2018, he said, the Positive Link program was just for Monroe County. "I was able to see what a gem it was and how fantastic it was. We were able to make contacts in 42 other counties and expand the program's influence and impact," he said.

The program's goal is to reduce emergency room visits, help stop the disease, provide psycho-social support with counseling and social services and help with supportive housing, he explained. Since he arrived, a clinic was opened here with a nurse practitioner who sees patients and provides them medical support.

"It's just an incredible thing we do that no one knows about," Shockney said. "I have not been a part of an organization that has dedicated the level of resources to a community as much as IU Health."

He also commended the support of the Monroe County Health Department, which reached out to the hospital in the late 1960s to help provide county health nurse support. Now, he added, the public health nurses are employees of IU Health Bloomington and help with the Positive Link program.

Hospital Social Services Are Important
Connection to Community

When people stay at the hospital, they expect their medical problems to be treated. But many might not expect to receive help to readjust to their home situations and cope with changes in their lives due to their health conditions after leaving the hospital.

Becky Hrisomalos, a first-generation American raised by her Greek parents in South Bend, wanted to smooth that pathway back home for patients and ease their concerns after leaving the hospital, whether they visited the emergency room or stayed for a longer period due to a serious illness or injury.

She had the chance to do that under the leadership of Roland "Bud" Kohr, who was president of Bloomington Hospital from 1966 to 1995, after he established a Social Work Department soon after he arrived. Ruth Gray was the first director, and Hrisomalos said they, along with Judy Talley, worked to develop the department's services.

Hrisomalos, who graduated from IU with bachelor's and master's degrees in social work, said she found just the right place when she began working at the hospital as a social worker. "I have always loved working at the hospital. I also loved helping the medical community. I was a social worker by profession and my husband, Frank, was a physician, so I felt like the hospital was just perfect for me." Her husband for 64 years, a long-time Bloomington physician, passed away in 2015.

Hrisomalos, whose two sons are doctors and two daughters are dentists, worked at the hospital for 23 years, including 17 years as Social Work Department director, until she retired in the mid-1990s. She said the department would arrange for patients to receive home care, if needed, and set up any type of training at the hospital or near patients' homes if they lived out of town.

Becky Hrisomalos, worked at the hospital for 23 years, including 17 years as Social Work Department director, until she retired in the mid-1990s. She also developed and led the Meals on Wheels program. *Photo submitted by Becky Hrisomalos.*

"We helped them find home care in all different areas. We would search around and find some resources because people couldn't always come back to Bloomington. Sometimes they needed nursing visits, someone to check on their surgeries and to help them with the healing process," she explained. IU social work students often helped the department to make arrangements, she added.

If people needed follow-up visits, sometimes social workers would go to their homes to make sure they received good medical care and follow-up instructions from doctors, but also to make sure they had the basics, including proper food, transportation, and housing, said Hrisomalos, who was once named Region 6 Social Worker of the Year by the Indiana Chapter of the National Association of Social Workers.

She recalled also helping emergency room patients who wouldn't have anyone at home to help them or didn't know about resources in the community, so she would find them for the patients.

"We were really involved and happy to help and solve lots of problems and to help find the services they couldn't find themselves," said Hrisomalos, former president of the State Social Work Directors Association.

Now, these types of services for patients are provided by nurses and social workers in the hospital's Integrated Care Management Department, directed by Kathryn Bennett, a registered nurse. She became director in 1996, when the hospital combined the Social Work and Utilization Departments into one area with expanded duties.

"At around 1996–97, the patients we were discharging were much more medically complex, and the reasons for discharging to nursing homes, rehab hospitals, long-term acute care hospitals were due to complex medical needs more than social needs," Bennett explained. But the social workers' roles changed from discharge planning to providing social services to patients, as they are the experts on social assessments and needs, emotional support for patients and families, and cultural support for patients, added Bennett. "Their skills were much more needed for these patient needs than to arrange for nursing home admissions."

Bennett, a 30-year hospital employee, has seen the department grow with increasing needs of patients. The 20-member department now has four social workers, 12 registered nurse case managers, three case manager assistants, and one licensed practical nurse discharge advocate. They cover all medical and surgical units, the neonatal unit, and emergency services.

"Our department is very important to the patients and the community," she said. The staff's goal is to reduce hospital readmissions and provide a safe transition from hospital back into the community, she added.

"We provide post-hospitalization planning in a very medically complex system. We work with patients and families to help them understand their insurance benefits as it relates to post-discharge care. We also are important to the community, as we try to protect hospital resources by helping patients move through the system as efficiently as possible, allowing us to have the capacity to care for the new patient who has medical needs the hospital can provide."

*Meals on Wheels Has Been Providing
Healthy Food for Decades*

When Hrisomalos read an article in 1973 about a Meals on Wheels program in England, she said, she thought right away, "Oh, we ought to do that."

Then she did.

She got to work setting up the program in Bloomington, initially organized by the hospital's Social Work Department that she directed. Hrisomalos said the meal delivery program had just started on the East Coast in the US and also in a few places in central Indiana, which she visited.

She headed a committee that conducted surveys to gauge interest in starting Meals on Wheels and found positive reaction.

After organizers contacted local churches, home health care agencies, and civic clubs and spoke at many meetings, enough money was raised for food storage equipment and attorneys' fees to establish a not-for-profit organization, Hrisomalos said. She and four other women signed the document establishing the program.

The first meals were delivered on February 18, 1974, to four clients by three volunteers, according to the Meals on Wheels website.[3]

Hrisomalos said Meals on Wheels initially started for former hospital patients who needed certain diets, but it expanded to others who needed the service. "I knew there were people out there who needed some kind of support, like a sugar-free or low-residue diet, so the hospital could provide that," she said. "The doctors were very supportive of the program.

"People paid for the meals, except those who couldn't afford it. I had an arrangement with the hospital. We didn't turn anybody down, but most people did pay. The meals were made in the hospital cafeteria and at a nearby nursing home run by the Local Council of Women," she recalled.

"Our social workers loved going into the homes of people. It was wonderfully accepted," she said.

In 2010, Bloomington Meals on Wheels, Inc. hired its first paid executive director, Kathy Romy, who stayed until 2019, when Carrie McHaley became director. The organization forged a partnership with Bloomington Hospital Foundation in 2010 for fundraising and investment support to help eligible clients not able to pay for their meals. The meals, provided twice a day Monday through Friday under physicians' prescriptions, are still prepared at the hospital, as well as at Meadowood Retirement Community.

The number of volunteers who delivered meals and the homebound people who ask for them have grown over the years. As of 2020, more than 250 volunteers deliver more than 1,000 meals a month to 84 clients, according to the Meals on Wheels website. To get the service, clients must be unable to prepare their own meals due to chronic illness, advanced age, or disability, or due to recovery from hospitalization or illness.[4]

Hrisomalos said, at age 90, she still delivers meals with a partner, who shares driving duties with her. "It is a joy to know we could help people go home safely and to continue to get the right kind of food.

"I feel wonderful that God has allowed me to stay healthy enough that I can still help people," she added. "I have loved every minute."

Contributions Improved Some Public Health Outcomes

Bloomington Hospital, as an institution, has worked over the years to help create positive results in decreasing the teen pregnancy rate, smoking rates, and obesity rates, among other health outcomes.

Making a community-wide impact on improving public health outcomes is one of the toughest challenges facing any health care provider. Changing decades-old health behaviors, especially in a state consistently ranking in the lowest tier nationally of health outcomes, is a difficult endeavor, many health experts agree.

With all of the other factors influencing health behaviors and outcomes, health experts say it's hard to determine conclusive causes for advances in people's overall health. But Dr. James Laughlin, chief practice officer of IU Health Bloomington Hospital, said, "To some degree, I think you can make a link between the hospital's and local health providers' focus on certain public health problems and an improvement in those conditions."

It's clearly a team effort, though, involving local agencies, IU academic entities, and local physicians' groups, to develop programs and bring attention to health problems, he said.

"We've also developed very good partnerships with community resources, such as the Bloomington Community Foundation and Bloomington Health Foundation, to help provide some of these services," he said. "We have a lot of collaborative arrangements with IU School of Public Health and School of Nursing. We provide the patients for them and they provide some expertise, and we form these teams to provide services in the community."

The goal is making systemic changes.

"So the mission is to help improve the health and the community outside of the hospital as well, long-term. That's one of the things we're working on—taking what's working here and trying to expand that," said Laughlin, a 43-year practicing pediatrician specialist in pulmonology. He founded a pediatrics group, now part of a larger group called IU Health Southern Indiana Physicians.

Looking at health statistics for Indiana counties, Monroe County fares relatively well in some key areas, admittedly in a state where many health outcomes are among the lowest in the country. Overall, a 2019 county-by-county health rankings survey conducted by the Robert Wood Johnson Foundation listed Monroe County nineteenth among Indiana's 92 counties in health outcomes, ranging from infant mortality and low birthweight to diabetes prevalence. The county's overall ranking for health factors, including adult smoking, adult obesity, and teen births, was sixteenth of 92 counties.

Monroe County's adult smoking rate is 19 percent, compared to the state's rate of 21 percent. The county's adult obesity rate is 25 percent, compared to 33 percent for the state. The teen birth rate is 8 per 1,000 births, significantly lower than the state's rate of 28 per 1,000 births. And the county's life expectancy was nearly 80 years, almost three years higher than the state average of 77.1 years, the report said.[5]

Smoking Cessation Efforts

In the last five to 10 years, Laughlin said, the hospital has been intentionally developing a more regional approach to studying these statistics and dealing with outcomes. If you look at Monroe County, for example, he said the lower smoking rates aren't all due to the hospital's efforts, although it does have a very active smoking cessation program.

As part of the Monroe County Tobacco Coalition, educators provide "Beat Tobacco" cessation classes through the IU Health Community Health Department. The free classes at the hospital and its Community Health building offer options to help quit smoking, tips on battling side effects, and guidance and support from educators.

Weiss-Kennedy said the Community Health Department also offers a 1-800 support line and nicotine replacement therapy. While she said cigarettes are the big culprit, vaping is also causing problems. So, the department offers an educational, eight-week curriculum for vaping one evening a week, with help from the Monroe County Health Department.

Laughlin also explained his pediatric group was involved in a successful smoking cessation study with the Academy of Pediatrics for two years. "We intentionally talked to parents when they came in and asked if they would like help with stopping smoking. We were able to document in those patients that we studied a 25 percent reduction in smoking," he said.

"So, there is a lot of support for that," Laughlin added. "The question is how we get that expanded more outside of Bloomington, where the smoking rates are much, much higher."

The community impact was significant, too, of long-time hospital pathologist Anthony "Tony" Pizzo on the antismoking movement. Pizzo, who died in 2015 at age 93, proposed and pushed to reality one of the first laws banning smoking in public places in Indiana. He was a member of the Bloomington City Council, which passed the ordinance in 2003, after considerable controversy and debate.

Teen Pregnancy

For Weiss-Kennedy, one of the big success stories has been the drop in teen pregnancies in Monroe County. She said the rate of 8 out of every 1,000 teen girls getting pregnant is one of the lowest in the country, and some rates in nearby southern Indiana counties go up to 40 per 1,000.

"I really feel like that has been one of our shining stars," she said. The Community Health programs aren't the only reason, but they have to be helpful and have some effect, she added.

The programs offered in the school offer age-appropriate discussion about the risks of early pregnancy, how birth control works, and safe sexual practices. "It's all from the standpoint of health. No moral judgments are made. The curriculum is evidenced-based education," she said. "I think the forward-thinking by the schools to allow us to go into the schools and train teachers that has helped."

Weiss-Kennedy also mentioned that her department collaborates with schools, Purdue Extension, and the health department, to try to expand the reach to a larger population.

Obesity Management

The hospital also has been supportive of reducing obesity in the community.

"We have a program, GOAL—Get Onboard Active Living—which is a healthy lifestyles program that we have in place targeting high-risk families," said Laughlin. "It's also been expanded to the schools, where we have an after-school program."

He added, "It is a perfect example of a collaborative arrangement between IU Health Bloomington Hospital, our pediatric group, IU School of Public Health, IU School of Nursing, and the city parks department—all partners—to provide sites, services, and personnel to support this program."

GOAL, which is free to families with children ages 6 to 18, encourages healthy lifestyles through nutrition, behavior, and physical activity education. Children with body mass indexes at or above the 85th percentiles are referred by primary care physicians. The families receive education on maintaining a healthy, balanced diet, increasing physical activity, reducing sedentary behaviors, developing a positive body image, building stronger familial relationships, gaining confidence to try new foods, and overcoming obstacles to being active, according to the IU Health GOAL website.

GOAL 2.0 extends nutrition information from GOAL into an eight-week program with a registered dietitian. For four weeks, the dietitian provides hands-on cooking lessons with children and parents to teach meal preparation and involve the children.

During the remaining four weeks, families discuss meal planning, shopping on a budget, last-minute meals, and other topics for parents. Basic nutrition education activities are provided for children. The children also get group and one-on-one physical activity sessions, and the parents receive individualized health coaching.[6]

Programs like GOAL and other similar efforts, said Laughlin, help keep the public's focus on healthy lifestyles.

"Monroe County has one of the lowest obesity rates in the state. Is there a correlation? Maybe it's because Bloomington has more people who are more interested in being healthy," he said. "But I think this (program) complements that and provides resources for people that want to become healthier and fight that problem. I've always said you have to keep these things on the forefront of people's minds, and let them know that we, in the medical field, think it's important."

Overall, the hospital provides numerous free or service-type programs for chronic disease management to deal with obesity, smoking cessation, addiction services, and behavioral health services, Laughlin said. Many of them don't generate revenue for the hospital, but cost the hospital, although grants help support the costs, he explained.

"There are a lot of things we're wanting to do to partner with community partners to be able to provide the resources and support for (people) to have a good result," said Laughlin. He mentioned a national electronic platform, called Aunt Bertha, which was started within IU Health in mid-2020.

The site provides people with health-related resources, on a county-by-county basis, with which they can link electronically or get appointments to visit, he explained. The services can help people with diabetes, smoking cessation, exercise, and many other needs. Physicians can use it to find resources for their patients and the public can access it on their own.

CERTIFICATIONS AND DESIGNATIONS SHOW
HOSPITAL MEETS HIGH STANDARDS

Many local residents and even patients may know little about IU Health Bloomington Hospital's certifications and designations—and even less about how earning them positively influences the quality of care they receive.

"Health care is a highly credentialed and regulated industry," said Shreve, former member of the Bloomington Hospital board of directors. "There are these pretty objective benchmarks you have to have in place to be certified as X or Y. Level 3 trauma center designation and Magnet hospital designation and neonatal designation are ones that we achieved while I was on the board."

Overall, the hospital is accredited by the Joint Commission on Accreditation of Healthcare Organizations, and is the only acute care facility within Monroe County.

To gain the commission's accreditation means a hospital passes an objective evaluation process that helps health care organizations measure, assess and improve performance, according to the commission. "Joint Commission certification improves the quality of patient care by reducing variation in clinical processes. The Joint Commission's standards and emphasis on clinical practice guidelines help organizations establish a consistent approach to care, reducing the risk of error," says the commission's website.[7]

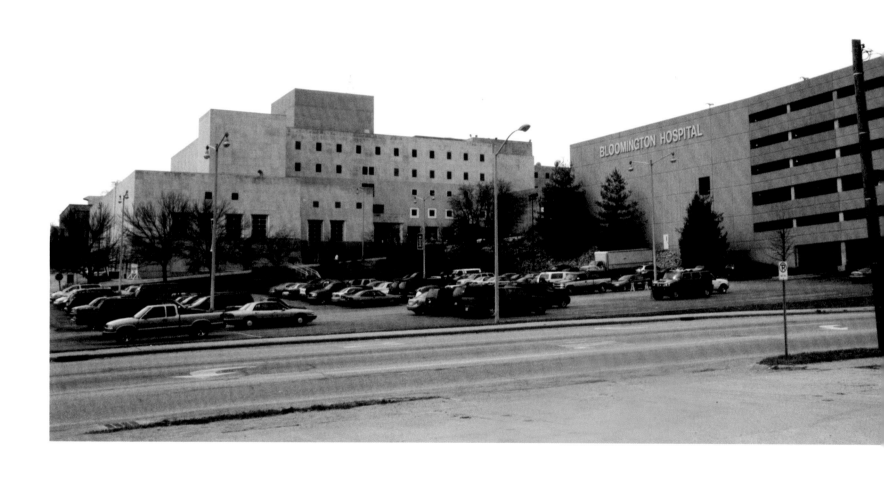

Bloomington Hospital exterior building shot taken in winter of 2003 with Second Street visible. *Photo credit: Monroe County History Center Photo Collection, Bloomington, Indiana.*

It took many years of effort, two lactation consultants, supportive local agencies—and a soft-spoken, harmonica-playing pediatrician to get Bloomington Hospital designated as a "baby-friendly" hospital under an international program.

"We worked on it for a long time and finally earned it in 2011," said Dana Watters, long-time Bloomington Hospital nurse, administrator and director of the IU Health Regional Center for Women and Children when the designation was earned. She retired as director in 2015.

The World Health Organization (WHO) and UNICEF launched the Baby-Friendly Hospital Initiative to help motivate facilities providing maternity and newborn services worldwide to implement the "Ten Steps to Successful Breastfeeding." Hospitals have to prove they're implementing the steps.

Among other actions, the designation requires hospitals to support and educate mothers on the importance of breast-feeding; help mothers immediately start the practice in the hospital; enable mothers and babies to room-in 24 hours a day; discuss the importance of breast-feeding with pregnant women; counsel mothers on the use and risks of using bottles and pacifiers; and to not provide breast-fed babies any food or fluids other than breast milk, unless medically indicated, according to the tensteps.org website.[8]

To get the designation, hospitals also cannot accept free or low-cost breastmilk substitutes, feeding bottles or teats. Watters explained that change had financial considerations because for many years baby formula companies gave free formula samples to the hospital, which would then give them to all new mothers. The hospital agreed in the early 2000s to stop accepting free formula, but then it had to purchase formula given only to mothers who definitely wanted to use it, she said.

WHO's research showed, Watters explained, that hospitals that paid for formula were more likely to actively support breast-feeding for its new mothers.

Bloomington Hospital's effort started with a neonatal nurse who became a lactation consultant with a certification in breast-feeding, and then another lactation consultant helped advance the process, Watters said. Staff at Women, Infants and Children, an agency supporting mothers and young children, and doctors' offices with lactation consultants also have helped lactating moms, she added. The Bloomington Area Birth Services, a nonprofit organization which had a lactation center supporting breast-feeding women, assisted, too, Watters said. (The agency closed in 2015, but continued to offer some classes for expectant mothers.)

"We were able to build an RN-nurse base here with these two individuals, particularly, who pushed and shoved to bring us where we needed to be with lactation consulting," she said.

Watters gave credit to Dr. Richard K. Malone, a pediatrician affiliated with Southern Indiana Physicians-Riley Physicians Pediatrics. "Dr. Malone was essential to the hospital going toward baby-friendly designation. He did that by talking to other physicians and carrying the message to them. He kept all the docs understanding the important of breast-feeding. They trust each other and listen to each other," said Watters, who recalled his harmonica playing.

He and the two lactations consultants, for example, stressed not sending formula home with mothers. "Science shows that moms are more likely to stop breast-feeding if you send home fancy little packages of formula," Watters said. "It's not good practice to do that."

One of the outcomes of this effort is that nurses had to care for both mothers and babies together.

"That was a unique change from providing separate care to caring for both. There was a whole new set of skills nurses had to learn," she said. "It was a national trend to care for them together, and it makes more sense for the patient. But it was a very difficult transition for nurses in all hospitals."

Magnet Nursing Designation Earned and Nursing Expertise Advances

With advances in technology and doctors learning new specialties, the nurses were expected to learn more and perform more complicated tasks.

"We've opened an open heart service and a cardiac cath lab. We opened a critical care unit and began performing taking care of patients with craniotomies," said Debra S. Wellman, hospital associate chief nursing officer-practice. "When you change those types of services, you must also increase the nursing staff and their level of expertise."

"We have an amazing critical care for our neo-natal babies. Over the years, we have continued to create specialty services ... Each one of those continues to challenge us to elevate the practice of nurses and their education and knowledge," stressed Wellman, an IU Health Bloomington Hospital nurse, educator and leader for 45 years. She also recalled when the hospital started doing neuro-surgery and vascular surgery.

To keep nurses up-to-date, the hospital has done training in the facility and sent many nurses to other hospitals, particularly IU Health Methodist and University Hospitals, to learn how to assist with the open heart program. In addition, pediatric nurses were sent to Riley Hospital for Children at IU Health to learn about neonatal critical care.

But the biggest accomplishment in terms of nursing training and preparedness occurred the first time in 2010 when the hospital achieved the "Magnet" designation from the American Nurses Credentialing Center, part of the American Nurses Association (ANCC). The hospital was re-designated in 2014 and in 2020.

"That's a big milestone," said Wellman, who said the initial effort took two years to complete. "Only 7 percent of hospitals nationally are Magnet designated, so it's a very prestigious accomplishment."

The American Nurses Association created a nursing excellence blueprint, called Magnet, which recognizes hospitals for their quality outcomes, their nurses' impact and influence, and educational accomplishments, she said.

"It seeks to recognize hospitals that acknowledge and utilize their registered nurses and their team members in achieving good outcomes," she said. When I assumed director's position for nursing, I was also the Magnet program director and helped the hospital move toward that designation."

Wellman taught for nine years in the IU School of Nursing but still worked part-time at the hospital as a patient care director. "I am so passionate about nurses and the power and influence they have that I came back to the hospital full-time to be a part of that (Magnet) journey. I was like, 'woo, sign me up, I want to be a part of that.'"

She said the nursing staff really focused on helping licensed practical nurses to become registered nurses and on registered nurses with associate degrees to become baccalaureate-trained registered nurses. Financially, the hospital supported the effort through offering tuition-reimbursement and flexible schedule to allow nurses to attend classes during the day, she added.

"We focused a lot on the education and growth of our nurses in relation to becoming a Magnet hospital. Those are ways we supported our staff to go back to school and accomplish their educational accomplishments," said Wellman. She started as a licensed practical nurse and earned a bachelor's degree in nursing and a master's degree in nursing administration.

But getting that designation took a lot of work.

"During that time frontline nurses became 'Magnet champions' who worked collaboratively with nursing leadership to review and verify we were poised to meet the ANCC Magnet components," said Wellman. "We reviewed patient satisfaction and quality outcomes and created shared governance structures to assure nurses and other clinicians implemented best practices for patient care."

Yet they also enjoyed the journey.

Wellman said nurses had fun hosting competitions to disseminate information about our journey through poster contests to show why they are Magnet nurses and creating poems and songs to illustrate the meaning of the designation.

The document submitted was 3,000 pages long. Three American Nurses Association made a site visit lasting three days in 2009. "It was a stressful, yet exhilarating three days as we escorted the surveyors around our organization. They were very impressed with our engaged staff and the many great quality outcomes our teams were achieving through their practice."

Their hard work paid off.

Now, 62 percent of the hospital's nurses have bachelor's degrees in nursing, compared to 36 percent in 2009, Wellman said. The Institute of Medicine's "call to action" wants hospitals to have 80 percent registered nurses at the minimum of the baccalaureate level. "The institute showed that patients' mortality increased and outcomes improved as the nurses' education increased," she said.

Watters, retired director of the IU Health Regional Center for Women and Children, said research also has shown common practices exist that lead nurses to want to be hired at certain hospitals related to safety, education, and utilization of evidence-based practices. "It is an environment where you want to work and there's respect between nurses, nurse leaders and administrator leaders," she stressed.

To earn the Magnet designation, Watters said, the hospital has to submit documents showing its policies and allow nursing association officials to visit the hospital and interview nurses. The hospital has to pay certain fees, tuition reimbursement, and resources for nurses to do medical research on best practices.

"It's an expensive and lengthy process, so the hospital administration has to support it financially and in theory," she said.

Wellman clearly remembered the relief and happiness the staff felt the day the hospital first received word it earned the designation.

"I was out of town on vacation and was with my family at the beach calling in to a packed Wegmiller Auditorium. Every seat was filled by Bloomington Hospital team members across all disciplines and specialties awaiting to hear the results of our Magnet designation quest," she said.

"When the Magnet program analyst shared the news about our first Magnet designation, the crowd erupted in cheers and celebratory hugs and high fives. I was dancing on the beach and celebrating with my family," said Wellman. "This was a great day in the life of our organization, as it truly was an award which reflected our team member's passion, commitment, and dedication to each other and those we are privileged to serve."

The Magnet designation is a plus, Watters explained, because when nurses look for positions, the Magnet designation tells them the hospital has met very stringent criteria and inspection. "For nurses, it tells them this is a place they want to work. You create an environment where nurses don't want to leave. This helps with recruitment and retaining nurses."

Watters also speaks about the hospital's educational support from personal experience. She earned a master's degree in nursing from Indiana Wesleyan University, which was allowed to offer classes at Bloomington Hospital. In addition, IU and Ivy Tech Community College also provided classes at the hospital, and practicing nurses came here for clinical experience, she said. Nurses at the hospital and people the community are open to take the courses.

"It's good business," said Watters. "There's a nursing shortage and it's going to get worse. It's smart for a hospital to embrace whatever they can to have educational programs within the community."

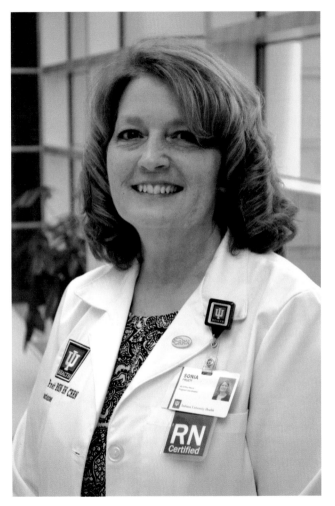

Sonia Pruett is the coordinator of the IU Health Bloomington Hospital stroke center, which has been certified as a primary stroke center since 2007. *Photo submitted by Sonia Pruett.*

Certified Stroke Center Provides Treatment and
Recovery Support

When people in this area have strokes, they can be assured that IU Health Bloomington Hospital has the resources and expertise to give them the care and treatment they need, according to stroke center coordinator Sonia Pruett. The fact the hospital has been certified as a primary stroke center every two years since 2008 is a key indication of its quality, she said.

"We are one of the few certified stroke centers in southern Indiana, and there are no other stroke certified hospitals in our surrounding counties," said Pruett. Nationally, she added, the certification isn't rare, but the designation shows the public the hospital meets all the national requirements for a stroke center related to staffing, treatment, and education outside and inside the hospital.

The Joint Commission on Accreditation of Healthcare Organizations, a national accrediting body, awards the certifications. More than 1,000 hospitals throughout the country are certified primary care stroke centers in all 50 states.

"You have to have a certain number of patients and meet percentages for standard of care," said Pruett, a nurse practitioner who has been stroke coordinator since 2015. "The commission recertifies hospitals every two years to make sure we're doing everything we say we're doing."

She gave a lot of credit to registered nurse Susan Savastuk, the hospital's first stroke program coordinator. She started working on getting certification with a group of people a few years before the designation was awarded.

"It was one of those things I knew I wanted to do because of her," said Pruett. "She built it from nothing."

To earn the designation, hospitals have to have a dedicated stroke-focused program, staffed by qualified medical professionals trained in stroke care, according to the Joint Commission's website. The hospital also must demonstrate it provides individualized care to meet stroke patients' needs and use data to assess and continually improve the quality of care for stroke patients.

A primary stroke center must be able to treat patients with ischemic (blood vessel blockage types of stroke) using a clot-busting drug, the commission states. A comprehensive stroke center, though, also must be able to treat such patients with catheter-based procedures to remove blood clots, as well as provide neurosurgical services for stroke patients. Indianapolis and a few other cities in Indiana have comprehensive stroke centers at hospitals.[9]

Pruett explained that IU Health Bloomington Hospital works closely with other hospitals in the area to accept patients for treatment. About 300 people annually have strokes in the hospitals 11-county area, but some stay at their local hospitals.

"If they get the clot-busting medicine, they have to come to a stroke center. There are pretty strict criteria for managing them after they get the medicine because they are at a high risk of bleeding," she said.

While no treatment existed for hundreds of years for a stroke, now hospitals can administer alteplase, a clot-busting drug, if patients make it to the hospital within a certain period of time, she said. The drug will break up the blood clot and restore blood to the brain, eliminating or lessening the severity of consequences.

The in-patient rehabilitation available at the hospital has been a huge benefit to patients, she said. "Having that acute care at our hospital is a big part of stroke rehabilitation. The sooner patients do that, the better off they are," she said.

Pruett also stressed that representatives from every unit of the hospital, including the emergency department, neurology, intensive care, and the ortho-neuro unit, support the work of the stroke center. "There is a mountain of people behind me to make sure we are providing that care on the floor every day."

She also emphasized the stroke center focuses a lot on preventative care and education in the community by sending staff to nursing homes, schools, health fairs, farmers' markets, county fairs, and other sites, and talking on radio programs, even sponsoring billboards.

"We don't want people to have a stroke, so we do a lot of stroke prevention education," Pruett said. She said the center keeps track of where their patients live and if more stroke patients come from a particular county, then more education efforts are directed there.

"The plan is to get them to cut their risk," said Pruett. "We talk about good diets and exercise—at least 30 minutes a day. We talk about low-fat diets. We talk about how to recognize the signs and symptoms of a stroke and the need to call 911 first."

Pruett emphasized the center has developed a stroke support group that meets monthly and regularly attracts a small core group of people, plus others who come occasionally. Often, speakers, such as pharmacists, lawyers, and health care providers, will address the group, and members will help each other find solutions to problems or resources.

"It's more about identifying the barriers they have in their lives and helping them to cope with them and navigating some of the things that go along with aging," said Pruett. "Many have significant disabilities for the rest of their lives."

Hospice Care Helps People Die with Dignity

Ellen Surburg remembers the time, decades ago, when hospice care was a scary thought.

"Hospice as a concept has gained acceptance over the years. When I started, it was a scary thought. But has been accepted more and more, as more and more families needed it," said Surburg, a registered nurse and former director of the Hospice of Bloomington.

She was among a small group of concerned citizens responsible for starting hospice care here. They formed a non-profit organization in 1979 to "bring comfort to patients who were otherwise dying alone in the hospital," she said. Hospice of Bloomington became a department of Bloomington Hospital in 1987 under the leadership of director Carol Ebeling. Currently, Stephanie Cain is the regional director of IU Health Home Care and Hospice.

Surburg said a community fundraising and bereavement program, called Light Up A Life, began in 1987 that benefited hospice services. Hrisomalos, who directed the hospital's social work department, was instrumental in initiating this program, she said. Gifts from individuals were given in honor or in memory or to celebrate a significant person. Names of those honored were posted on a lighted case on the city's Courthouse Square next to a Christmas tree.

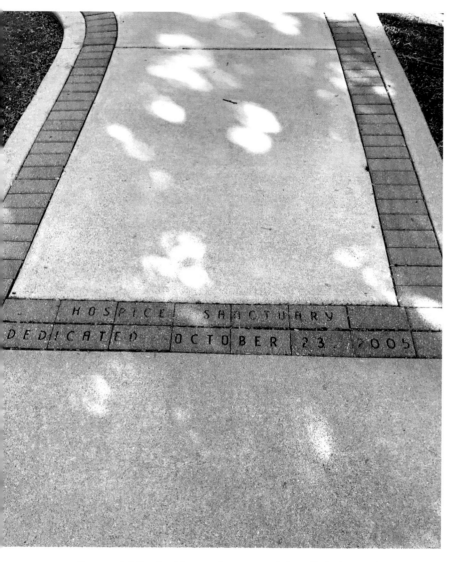

Centennial Garden Hospice Sanctuary: Sidewalk dedicated for Hospice Sanctuary in 2005. *Photo credit: IU Health Bloomington Hospital.*

A big goal of the new hospice department, Surburg explained, was to become certified in order to provide assistance with Medicare funding. In 1990, a team assembled to go through the certification process required by Medicare. In addition to Surburg, that group included volunteer physicians led by Pizzo, director of the hospital's pathology department; hospital chaplain John VanderZee; social worker Teresa Creek.

Medicare certification was accomplished in 1991. Surburg said that until that time, the hospital could only provide volunteer supportive care, but it couldn't provide nursing home visits without Medicare certification.

Surburg started working at the hospital in 1981 as a nurse. "I was aware of hospice, and I liked the concept," she recalled. When the position was available for a nurse to help the hospice get Medicare benefits, she sought that work. In 1990, she became acting hospice director and served as department director from 1995 until 2011, when she retired.

She learned early that hospice work appealed to her.

"I never avoided treating dying patients," Surburg said. "It was meaningful for me to work with the family and the patient. The whole spiritual aspect is rewarding. In my role, it was to support every aspect of the team.

"I wish I had started it so much earlier," Surburg said.

Hospice care was initially provided to patients in Monroe and parts of surrounding counties within a 25 mile-radius. The care was given to patients in more than a dozen long-term care facilities in the service area, meeting the goal of providing care to patients wherever they live, she said. Patients also were hospitalized when needed.

In the hospice model of care, she explained, patients received medical care from their own physicians. Dr. Brad Bomba Jr. became hospice medical director, leading the interdisciplinary team in delivery of hospice care. He now serves with Dr. Robert Stone, a palliative care physician who is associate director.

In the early 2000s, a transitions program was developed to provide support and comfort to patients who did not meet Medicare's criteria for coverage, said Surburg. This transitions program was a precursor to the palliative care program that followed.

Hospice was considered a major step forward that provided a new type of care for people in the last days of the lives. The seeds of the project emanated from a meeting between Surburg and Christopher Molloy, president of the Bloomington Hospital Foundation, a philanthropic organization that raised funds for hospital facilities, equipment and programs.

Surburg said Molloy visited hospital department heads looking for ways the foundation could help. She told him about the program's need for a hospice house. "The truth is he needed a project, and I had one," she recalled.

"It was amazing," she said of the foundation's major fundraising campaign that began in 2009. Within 18 months, $3 million was raised from the community. In planning for hospice house, she visited about a dozen of them around the country and worked with two architectural firms. "I wanted our hospice to look like a house, a Craftsman-style home built for hospice," she said.

The 10,000-square-foot hospice house was dedicated in October 2011. Now called the IU Health Bloomington Hospital Hospice House, the home is nestled on a three-acre wooded tract just south of Bloomington at 2810 S. Deborah Dr. It can accommodate 12 patients at a time and offers space for family members and friends to spend as much time as they want there.[10]

"The house was really designed to carry out the goals of hospice," said Surburg. "Families are encouraged and feel welcome there. Living areas are there where families can find solitude or find time together."

Hospice care is available 24 hours a day, seven days a week, to anyone facing a life-limiting illness with an expectancy of six months or less to live. Patients in the Hospice House can get the same high-level care they get in the hospital with around-the-clock nursing and services from a hospice medical director, social worker, and chaplain, she said.

But the majority of hospice care is given to patients in their homes with individualized services that include pain and symptom management, often referred to as "comfort care," according IU Health Hospice website. The main goal, the website says, is to provide compassionate care that meets the emotional, spiritual and physical needs of patients facing the end of life.[11]

Home Health Care Provides Unique Services

Nurse administrator Eleanor Rogers was on the front lines of the evolution of public health nursing and home health care in Bloomington for decades. With hospital stays decreasing in length, home care has become more and more important to the community.

She spent some 25 years with the Indiana Public Health Nursing Association in Monroe County, starting as a visiting nurse, then as supervisor of the nursing staff and as director. After the agency merged with Bloomington Hospital's Home Health Care in the late 1980s, she became vice president of public health, retiring in 2010.

Overall, the goals of the association and the hospital's program were similar: Provide public health services, either in homes, schools and other settings, and education to help the community live healthier.

From her vantage point, Rogers said the hospital and her department responded well to public health concerns and individuals' health care needs that could be taken care of in homes.

"The hospital has always had its finger in things that needed to be done," said Rogers, 80. "We were all pretty well versed in what was going on. Sometimes we started things on our own, and sometimes people came to us and said, 'Isn't there something you can do about this?'"

Rogers, who came to Bloomington in 1977 when her husband, Kenneth, became IU director of international services, said the nursing association and hospital worked well together even before the merger. Nurses from the association talked to Home Health Care about which of the hospital's patients needed help at home after being released.

"There were a number of underinsured, uninsured people in the community who were not getting the health care they needed," Rogers stressed.

Over the years, she said the nursing association took on a number of public health needs: childhood immunizations, sexually transmitted diseases, children with low birth weights, people with AIDS/HIV, and the WIC program. The hospital's Community Health Department later took over some of those responsibilities, including WIC and working with people with AIDS/HIV in its Positive Link program, Rogers said.

The merger helped improve services, as the popularity of home health care grew. "We had greater access to people who needed assistance at home after the merger," she said. "At that point, a lot of hospitals decided they wanted to have a home health care program."

Rogers said the Health Services Bureau operated for a period of time to take people of need and get them referred to physicians who were willing to give them free care. Out of that effort came the Community Health Access Program, known as CHAP, a community-wide clinic.

"It was an effort to provide health care, but we emphasized what nurses and social workers could do for people. We started only with nurse practitioners, although the needs were greater than what the nurses could do," she explained. "There was an understanding with local physicians. Any private physician who would take a referral would get $10 a visit. The hospital would provide us with medication and diagnostic testing for patients."

Now, CHAP is one of a small number of clinics statewide that offers medical care to indigent and uninsured patients without federal funding.

After she retired, Rogers said she was asked to serve on the board of the Local Council of Women, the organization that started the hospital. Since she became council board president, she automatically got a position on the Bloomington Hospital board of directors and served when the hospital decided to join IU Health in 2010. She served on the hospital board until it was dissolved when the IU Health South Central Region board was created.

Currently, the IU Health Bloomington Home Care team members, are under the guidance of Cain, regional director of

IU Health Home Care and Hospice. Home care services are available 24 hours a day, seven days a week, from a wide range of professionals. They include registered nurses, home health aides, physical and occupational therapists, speech and language pathologists, medical social workers, dietitians, pharmacists, and respiratory therapists.

People can qualify for home care services if they have one of a number of conditions, such as Alzheimer's disease, cancer, diabetes, heart failures, stroke, infection, and joint replacement. They can get help managing medications, monitoring lab tests, caring for wounds, giving infusions and tube feedings, preventing falls, rehabilitating from strokes, and other types of care.

IU Health Olcott Center for Cancer Education
Offers Support and Information

The experiences of long-time Bloomington civic leader Joan Olcott when she had breast cancer had a great impact on establishing a cancer education center here.

"How I wish there had been such a place when I was dealing with breast cancer," wrote Olcott, a two-time breast cancer survivor, in a handwritten note to IU Health nurse navigator Julie Darling in 2018.

Olcott was referring to the Olcott Center for Breast Health, which opened in Bloomington Hospital's Medical Arts Building in 1998. She and her husband, Lloyd, both of whom have died, donated a major contribution of $50,000 to help create that center. Darling was writing an article for the Olcott Newsletter on the twentieth anniversary of the center.[12]

The couple's contribution added to a campaign started by local breast cancer survivors and other concerned citizens who raised $35,000. To help with funding, the hospital enlisted the aid of the Hopewell Circle, named after the family who owned the farmhouse and property that was the location of the first hospital.[13]

In her letter, Olcott explained her background and life with her husband and the impetus for the donation. She wrote she was diagnosed with breast cancer in 1966 and had surgery and radiation. About the same time, she said, the hospital was considering some type of source or center "where women could receive information, support and encouragement during their cancer treatment."

That's what she said she would have liked while she had breast cancer. She expressed her gratitude for women who thanked her for the center. "I have received many verbal and written 'thank-yous' through the years from grateful women," she wrote. "I always say, 'Don't thank me. It is those wonderful, compassionate nurse navigators who have been so caring in your behalf.'"[14]

In March 2020, Joan passed away after a stroke. For many years, she had been a volunteer at the hospital and a member of the Bloomington Hospital Foundation and other community groups. Lloyd, who died in 2001, was a local businessman and long-time civic leader who served on the Bloomington Parks and Recreation Board, Bloomington City Council, and many other bodies.

The center, directed by Terri Acton, has since been renamed the IU Health Olcott Center for Cancer Education to reflect an expanded mission.

The center offers an extensive lending library, weekly support groups, genetics education, patient advocacy, art therapy, wig fittings, breast prosthetics fittings, and some individualized financial assistance. Free educational talks and materials are available to groups, schools, businesses, and individuals. Oncology

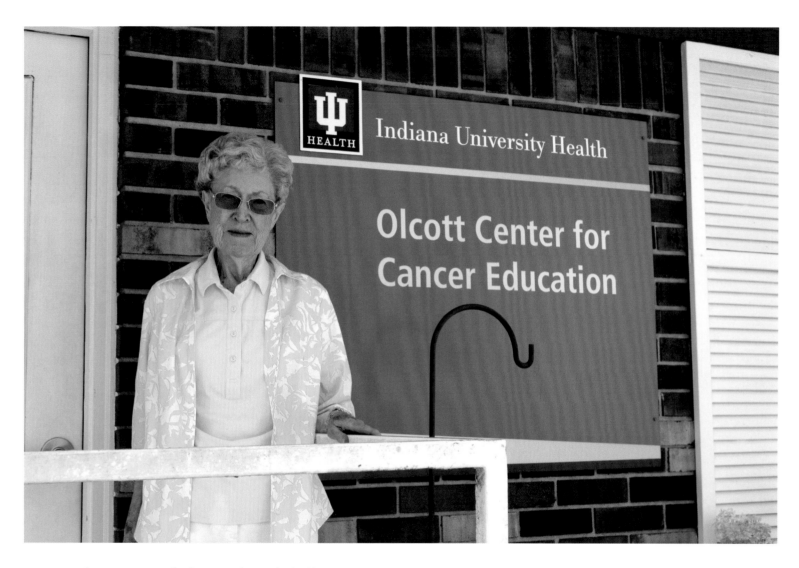

Long-time Bloomington civic leader Joan Olcott, who had breast cancer in 1966, and her husband Lloyd made a major contribution of $50,000 to establish the Olcott Center for Breast Cancer, which opened in Bloomington Hospital's Medical Arts Building in 1998. The center was later renamed the IU Health Olcott Center for Cancer Education. *Photo credit: IU Health Bloomington Hospital.*

certified, registered nurse educators provide one-on-one education with clients and their family members. All the services are free to anyone living in south central Indiana.[15]

Bloomington Health Foundation
Makes Significant Impact

For more than 55 years, an active philanthropic nonprofit organization of staff and volunteers has contributed to some of Bloomington Hospital's greatest needs in a myriad of ways.

Bloomington Hospital Foundation ceased operation in 2018, when the fundraising arm for IU Health Bloomington Hospital became the IU Health Foundation. Bloomington Health Foundation formed as a separate organization focusing on health needs of the community, including but not limited, to the hospital.

The independent foundation was established in 1965 with $3,000 in its treasury, as part of the Local Council of Women, according to the foundation's website. By the mid-1970s, the number of donors totaled more than 725, and Barry K. Hurtt was hired as the first director.

Initially, the foundation raised money for major equipment needs, including patient monitoring equipment for the intensive care unit, operating room equipment, and funds for a new telemetry system for the emergency room. It also donated almost $192,000 in 1982 to the hospital's expansion. Beginning in 1984, all major proposals for funding went through the foundation's board of directors, which includes community and health care leaders, the website says. Cook Group made major donations in the 1980s for innovations, including the Cook Cardiac Catheterization Laboratory.

The foundation and its donors continued in the 1990s to fund equipment needs, such as a transport incubator for obstetrics, Med Alert bracelets for hospice patients, and a transport monitor for the emergency department. It also funded the Adult Day Center and contributed $350,000 for the Healthmobile.

In 2000, the foundation organized the inaugural Hoosiers Outrun Cancer run-walk event, which raised $1 million that year and continues to be a big annual fundraiser. Funds also were raised in the 2000s for a helipad; a renovated catheterization lab; the Tichenor Fund for Children's Therapy, which funds equipment and resources for children with special needs; the in-patient Hospice House; and upgrades to the neonatal intensive care unit.

In 2014, the foundation's Trauma Campaign raised $320,000 to provide critical improvements to the hospital's trauma department. As a result, the hospital later earned a Level III Trauma Center designation.[16]

Over the decades, doctors and other health care providers, as well as patients, have benefited from the foundation's efforts and the community's financial backing.

Dr. James LaFollette, a long-time family practitioner who retired in 2009 from Southern Indiana Physicians, observed the impact the foundation's effort made over the years, especially in funding important medical equipment. He explained that having up-to-date equipment for doctors helps attract specialists, who improve health care and benefits provided to the community.

"When you have that equipment, you have a pretty big drawing area," he said. "It started in the 1970s. The Bloomington Hospital Foundation had a lot to do with all of this."

The hospital's programs and staff and affiliated organizations have made countless contributions to the community's health and well-being. Innovative changes to services and procedures, medical advancements, new equipment, and updated facilities all have influenced care for patients, access to health care, and good health outcomes.

Less visible are the daily actions and deeds of health care providers who step up when they see a need or a gap in services or even an individual or group of people who aren't being served as well as they could be.

Doctors, nurses, administrators and other providers are often in positions to see health and other types of needs of their patients and people in the community. Some have said they believe it's their duty to respond. Sometimes, they feel it's their responsibility, too, to help train younger people who are going to become doctors or nurses or give advice or encouragement to those thinking about getting into medicine.

In his 40 years as a family practitioner in Bloomington, LaFollette has seen many of those moments—and participated in them, as well. He considers himself fortunate to have practiced here, using hospital resources for some of his patients, and assisting in surgeries for his patients mostly during the first 20 years of his practice.

"Bloomington has been a great place for me to practice," said LaFollette, who came to Bloomington in 1969 and practiced with Dr. Charles McClary for 33 years. LaFollette said he had a large pediatric practice, delivered more than 1,000 babies, assisted in some 1,000 surgeries, and performed a lot of orthopedics work.

As a volunteer, he taught prenatal classes because he said he wanted young mothers to be well informed. Early in his practice, he talked with women involved in the La Leche League, a non-profit organization that supports breast-feeding. LaFollette said he also liked to help teach medical students, particularly to help them learn to do patients' medical histories and physical exams.

"I always had students in the office," he said. "My office was pretty much an open door for education." He also went to high schools and sometimes even elementary schools to explain the role of doctors.

"I felt like it was my responsibility," said LaFollette.

But he stressed that many doctors in Bloomington feel a similar strong obligation to improve health care in the community. He pointed to Pizzo for his antismoking efforts and to Rink for his drive to improve cardiovascular practices.

One effort he remembered most was taking care of indigent patients—and the help he received from other doctors and the hospital to do that.

"If I had a patient who was indigent and had to put them in the hospital, I didn't have any trouble getting a specialist to come see them," he said. "Parts of the community were really poor. If I needed help, I was able to find a specialist and the other doctors had to do it gratis, too. The hospital admitted them if they couldn't pay. I felt good that I could get to admit them."

Looking back, LaFollette said he appreciated all the support he received from the hospital for enabling him to expand his services, such as taking care of his patients in intensive care and assisting in surgery, as long as he remained up-to-date in his education.

Coyne, IU Health South Central Region board member, also recognized the hospital's role in supporting doctors and bringing high-level sophisticated care closer to this community. As an example, he mentioned the neonatal intensive care unit that allows mothers to get the care they need here for premature babies and those who need critical care.

"The babies' chances of survival and getting better quicker, being treated quicker, and therefore not having more significant consequences, were greatly enhanced over the years by advancements at the hospital," Coyne said.

But he thinks people sometimes take this type of care for granted. "It's hard for them to grasp. It takes so much to put that in place. That's what this hospital has done," Coyne said. "It's made this type of care available to so many more people in this region."

Taking a broad perspective, Peterson, chair of the IU Health South Central Region board, said the hospital and board members have to keep in mind their fundamental duties to the community and continue to ask themselves questions to make sure they're fulfilling those duties.

"Ultimately, our primary responsibility is to the citizens and patients in the communities and the regions. That's first and foremost in the front of everything we do. And first and foremost in

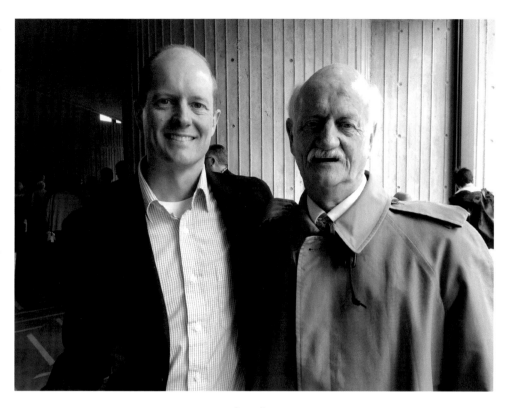

Dr. James LaFollette (right) a long-time family practitioner, who retired in 2009 from Southern Indiana Physicians, poses with his son, Dr. Chris LaFollette, who is a general practitioner in Bloomington. *Photo submitted by Dr. James LaFollette.*

the front of all of that is the quality of care we are delivering," he stressed.

"Are we delivering the right care at the right time? Do we have all the resources to do that? Do we have the systems and communication across all of that space well done?" he said, as questions that need to be answered all the time.

"We have to make sure," he stressed, "that the region and system are aligned, and we're all working together to take advantage of the power that a large, integrated health system can bring, more coordination throughout the system and the state of Indiana."

Tragic "Baby Doe" case puts hospital in national spotlight, leads to changes in ethics practices, federal rules

The brief life of "Baby Doe" in 1982 thrust Bloomington Hospital into a firestorm of debate and the national spotlight over parental rights to decide on lifesaving medical treatment for children born with disabilities.

"It was very traumatic over the six days the baby lived," recalled Dr. James L. Laughlin, a pediatrician who consulted with the Bloomington baby boy's pediatrician, Dr. James Schaffer. "There was a complete disagreement among the health care team about what to do."

Baby Doe, as he was named by the media, was delivered at the hospital on April 9 by obstetrician Dr. Walter Owens. Immediately after birth, the baby was found to have the features of Down syndrome and a birth defect causing part of his esophagus not to be connected properly with the stomach, said Laughlin.

Without surgery to correct his condition, called esophageal atresia, food wouldn't get to this stomach. So, he couldn't survive.

After health care providers disagreed and a court battle, the mother, 31, and father, 34, decided to withhold any lifesaving treatment or surgery. "So, the baby ended up dying, basically of starvation, because they (parents) wouldn't let the (hospital) put in an IV," said Laughlin, now chief practice officer for IU Health Bloomington Hospital.

The case, which received much national media attention, was debated among local citizens and the health care community here and elsewhere, and it particularly drew criticism from advocates of children with disabilities and right-to-life supporters. In the long run, the case had a broad impact on the way hospitals deal with disagreements over babies' treatment between parents and health care providers, and on the federal laws and rules regulating a child's care in similar cases.

"So, laws that were put in place were basically to protect disabled individuals and provide some protection for them through the government, regardless of the parents' decision," explained Laughlin. He added this case also led to hospitals developing multidisciplinary ethics committees to provide expert advice.

"They aren't a legal entity to say (what) has to be done, but to provide an outside opinion of what they would suggest," he explained.

Laughlin, a long-time pediatrician who founded Southern Indiana Pediatrics, said he was among several doctors who disagreed with the option Owens gave the parents to take no lifesaving steps and let the baby die. "The family was told by the obstetrician the baby would probably be severely retarded and always need help," remembered Laughlin.

The family physician, Dr. Paul Wenzler, who died in 1997, was upset by Owens' advice, Laughlin said. "So he consulted Dr. Schaffer, the couple's pediatrician, who consulted me because he wasn't getting anywhere. A number of us who were involved said we really don't know the extent of the baby's problems because they wouldn't let any tests to be done," he said.

Laughlin continued, "But our advice was that we need to have tests done, so we can make an informed decision about the extent of things that need to be done to treat the baby or not treat the baby . . . but they (parents) decided not to do that."

The case went through a series of legal steps, according to media reports. Families petitioned to adopt Baby Doe. A lawsuit was brought before Monroe Circuit Court Judge John Baker to require medical care. The parents testified they didn't believe babies with Down syndrome could lead very good lives. Owens spoke in defense of his advice to the parents. Laughlin, Wenzler, and Schaffer testified medical care should be provided for the baby at an Indianapolis hospital.[17]

Baker found that the parents "after having been fully informed of the opinions of two sets of physicians, have the right to choose a medically recommended course of treatment for their child in the present circumstances."[18]

Monroe County Prosecutor Barry Brown and Deputy Prosecutor Lawrence Brodeur, along with local attorney Philip Hill, selected by Baker as guardian ad litem for Baby Doe, filed a Child in Need of Services (CHINS) petition. The petition, supported by affidavits from Laughlin and Schaffer, argued the baby's life was endangered by his parents' refusal to provide necessary medical care.

But a Child Protection Committee from the Monroe County Department of Public Welfare concurred with the court's decision. Further requests to the Indiana Court of Appeals to review the decision and to the Indiana Supreme Court for emergency medical treatment also were denied. In a last ditch effort, Brodeur traveled on April 15 to Washington DC, where he planned to file an emergency petition before the US Supreme Court.[19]

But the baby's time had run out.

At 11 p.m., Baby Doe, named Walter by his parents after the obstetrician, died before the US Supreme Court could hear an appeal. Earlier that day, Schaffer and Laughlin made attempts in the hospital to try to give the baby intravenous feeding that were thwarted by Owens, who was watching over the baby, according to a series of articles, "The Death of Baby Doe," published on February 10, 1985, in the *Chicago Tribune*, written by Jeff Lyon. The articles said the doctors dropped efforts after another pediatrician examined the baby and said he was beyond recovery.[20]

"Ultimately," said Laughlin, "you want the parents to be able to provide those decisions, but it would have been nice to have been able to have more studies done so you knew what the problem was, and maybe have them see a geneticist and provide expert counseling so they could have made more of an informed decision."

But he recognized the problem of the health care team not agreeing on the best course. "That was the main issue. I think, most physicians believe the family should be the final voice in deciding these issues, and it shouldn't be taken out of their hands. But we also believe that they need to be informed appropriately to make a good decision."

Owens, who died in 2009 after a 42-year career practicing medicine, strongly felt the parents had the final voice in the Baby Doe case and, in general, individuals have the right to control their own health care decisions.

Owens explained his reasoning during testimony he gave in hearings in 1986 conducted by the administration of President Ronald Reagan, over this issue. "My conviction about the Baby Doe case was that this was a matter of personal liberty and family responsibility, and not something to be settled by me, the government, or anyone else," Owens said, according to an article on February 17, 1992, in the *Bloomington Herald-Times*.

"I feel that way with health care in general," he added in the article. "The individual has the right to as much information as can be produced to make his or her own decision."[21]

The impact of the baby's death and subsequent similar cases has affected, to a degree, the way hospitals handle these cases. Several years of controversy followed, during which lawyers, the public and medical experts debated the government's responsibilities and family or parental rights involved in these types of cases.

During the 1980s, a number of vocal advocates, including US Surgeon General C. Everett Koop, urged Congress to develop and adopt the Baby Doe amendment to the 1974 Child Abuse Prevention and Treatment Act. The amendment, passed in 1984, was the first attempt by the US government to directly intervene in treatment options for neonates born with severe congenital defects. This movement largely came about due to the Baby Doe case and another one called the Baby Jane Doe case involving a girl with spina bifida.

Under the Baby Doe rules, hospitals and physicians were told they must provide "maximal care to any impaired infant," except under select exceptions, as a requirement to receive federal funding, and they would be liable for medical neglect if they withheld treatment. Federal regulations were then issued that required hospitals to post public notices about reporting potential violations and setting up a telephone hotline to do so.

But many health care providers contended some of the rules were too intrusive and initiated a lawsuit that reached the US Supreme Court. In 1986, the court decided the anonymous hotline system was too intrusive, and the government could not intervene when a parent made the decision to withhold treatment, rather than the health care provider.

Instead, the Baby Doe rules transferred responsibility to hospital ethics boards and state child protective services agencies and instructed hospitals to set up reporting procedures, such the ethics panels, to quickly provide guidance and facts to parents.[22]

Under the rules, withholding treatment is only permissible if the newborn is irreversibly comatose, if treatment would only prolong its death, or if treatment would be inhumane, said the report "The Baby Doe Rules," published May 12, 2011, by the Embryo Project Encyclopedia, an international group of researchers who pursue goals related to the sciences of development biology and reproductive biology. Also, the report said the law holds that a physician's decision for neonatal care cannot be based on quality of life or other abstract concepts. If a case involves parents or their doctors choosing to withhold treatment, the report said, these review boards are obligated to inform child services as a potential instance of medical neglect.[23]

Laughlin said the Baby Doe case did make a positive change.

"Ethics committees were created, as a result of this case, and this led to these committees being standard at most health care systems and hospitals," said Laughlin. "Most hospitals didn't have ethics committees or anything set up to review cases like this when there's a discrepancy between family or parental decisions and physicians' or health care decisions."

Still, experts say medical and ethical communities are divided on how to respond to a parent's preferences to resuscitate or not resuscitate babies in distress.

In the years since Baby Doe and federal regulations, physicians have continued to withhold treatments, including life-sustaining medical treatments, from some newborns, said an article in the Georgia State University Law Review in 2009, called "The Aftermath of Baby Doe and Evolution of Newborn Intensive Care." One review of 165 deaths in the NICU at the University of California at San Francisco Medical Center from 1989 to 1992 showed 108 deaths resulted from withdrawing of life-sustaining therapy, according to the law review.

The review author, Mark R. Mercurio, said, "While neonatologists generally support the parental right to refuse treatment in certain situations, the threshold for that right appears to have moved." Specifically, he added in cases of babies with Down syndrome the standard of care for many years has been to provide surgical correction of intestinal atresias or heart disease, and parental refusal of such treatment would most likely be challenged in court and overruled.

But he also said the Baby Doe case could well be seen as good ethical reasoning—the parents' right to refuse treatment when the prognosis is extremely bleak—applied to bad data, as the quality of life for these babies was far less bleak than stated.[24]

5

EXTRAORDINARY CARE: MEDICINE FROM THE HEART

A FUNERAL, A FOOTBALL GAME, a baptism, a friendly chat, and even an offer to a patient's mother to practice giving shots on a nurse.

All of these scenarios are linked by one common thread—people caring for other people at the IU Health Bloomington Hospital over the past few decades.

In one case, nurses set up a funeral service in a hospital room for a patient who died unexpectedly and whose family couldn't afford one.

Another time, an intensive care team worked together for nearly a month to save a critically ill patient. She and her husband publicly thanked the staff during a high school football game he coached.

Years ago, a hospital employee arranged the baptism of a dying patient, who worked at the hospital, in the patient's home.

A hospital gift shop volunteer also chatted with a cancer patient who needed someone to talk to before going back to her room.

A nurse even volunteered to be injected with saline so a mother could practice before giving morphine shots to her terminally ill daughter at home.

Hospital staff and volunteers often perform acts of kindness outside of providing medical care. They extend thoughtful gestures, large and small, to put patients and family members at ease—sometimes in the last hours of life. Health care providers go above and beyond to save critically ill patients. And they work tirelessly, sometimes motivated by a desire to improve a health problem.

These deeds and special care aren't unusual at IU Health Bloomington Hospital now or in the past. Memories of these efforts stick with employees and volunteers years later, even after they have retired or now, as they move to the Regional Health Academic Center.

Certainly, people realize lives are saved and lost at hospitals and sometimes forever changed due to patients' health problems. Hospitals are unique places, where joy and sadness coexist. Health care providers and volunteers play a significant role in all of that.

THE BEST IN PEOPLE SURFACES

In a hospital setting, the best in people often emerges.

"Bloomington Hospital has had this long history of caring deeply about patients in their community and always wanting the best," said Lynn Coyne, local community leader and member of the IU Health South Central Region board of directors.

"They're (employees) always going to deliver the best care under whatever circumstances they're given. I saw that when I went to work as an orderly," he remembered from decades ago. "The heroic efforts the nurses would make to care for their patients was just amazing. I have such respect for them. It wasn't because they were being paid or whatever.

"People in health care care about what they do," Coyne continued. "They wouldn't be there if they didn't care because it's

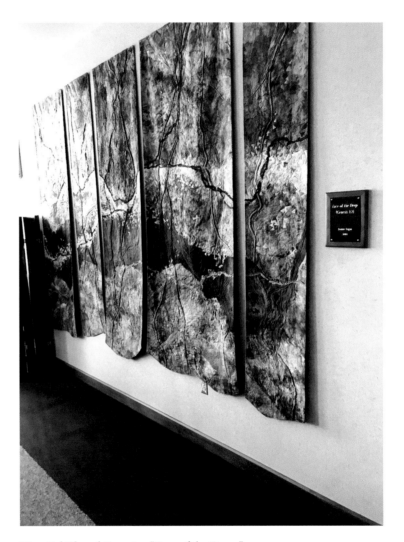

Hospital Chapel Tapestry "Face of the Deep."
Photo credit: IU Health Bloomington Hospital.

hard work. It's mentally hard, and your patients don't often like what you're doing."

Patty O. Booker, who previously was hospital educational services coordinator, cared deeply about a fellow employee and friend. She acted on that feeling when her friend, who was a terminally ill patient with cancer, needed her on December 30, 2002.

The patient had told her and two other employee friends that she was concerned about not being baptized but was reluctant to tell her husband and family.

"One day, her husband called me at work and said that she was at home and not doing well at all," recalled Booker, now project manager for hospital medical education. "I was at work when I got the call from him and some other employees within my department heard me tell her husband about her request to be baptized."

Booker wanted to arrange for her friend to be baptized, but she was concerned about getting her from her bed to the bathtub.

Her two employee friends and two paramedics helped make it happen. The paramedics overheard Booker talk about the problem of moving the woman from her bed. They volunteered to come to her friend's house and carried her on a sheet to the bathroom.

"I called the pastor at my church and asked if he could come and baptize her at home in the bathtub. Pastor Michael Douglas and his wife met us at my friend's house that day," Booker said.

"I can't tell you how much this meant to my friend and to all of us. Their generosity and support was very much appreciated," she stressed. "This was above and beyond the call of duty for them."

Booker's friend was baptized that afternoon. That evening, she passed away. "We all believed that was what she was waiting on," Booker said.

Sometimes small, simple gestures also can make a difference in patients' days or their frames of mind and let them know hospital employees care about them.

Jenny L. Gray, who serves as a patient account analyst, used to be a ward clerk on a small floor where patients stayed after leaving the intensive care unit. At that time in 1979, Gray took orders off the doctors' charts, changed the brown paper sacks taped to each patients' bed railings for their trash, and refreshed water pitchers.

"This was a fun time to get to know the patients on the floor and hear the stories of their lives and just get to know who I was helping take care of," Gray remembered.

She recalled one particular patient, a blind man, who had his service dog with him. But she said the patient wasn't well enough to walk his dog, and the nurses needed to care for patients. "So it was obvious I was the one who should do the job. The dog would just lay on his mat in the patient's room. I volunteered to walk his dog every evening at 10 p.m.

"Sometimes that wasn't so easy, as the dog was a large black Lab and he sometimes decided where HE wanted to go," Gray said.

Even taking the time for a few minutes of informal chatting can brighten a patient's day.

Mary Lou Foster, a 30-year employee who now is a physician biller/analysist with Revenue Cycle Services, said she volunteered at the hospital gift shop every second Thursday for seven years until 2002.

"I just really loved that gig," said Foster. "It was so awesome to get to be there for so many people, sometimes sharing in the celebration of a birth or mourning the loss of a loved one and, of course, waiting on an updated word from the outpatient surgery or emergency room, but mostly just letting visitors or family members take a break to browse and get a gift or a piece of candy."

One evening in 1999, a young adult woman came in pushing along her IV pole with her medications hanging from it. "You could tell that she was battling a serious illness, which turned out to be a cancer," Foster said. She was eating her lunch and immediately looked up when the woman came in and said she wanted to buy a gift. They found an appropriate gift and wrapped it together.

But the woman lingered.

"She wanted to stay for a bit before returning to her room. I was fine with that, so I just said 'of course, stay and hang out a bit,'" Foster said.

The two had a good conversation about a number of topics while Foster finished lunch. "I told her I was so sorry for her illness, and that I was praying for a positive outcome in her favor. She told me thanks for the help and for caring about her. We said good night and smiled, and I gave her a very soft hug."

Foster said she always remembered her and the 30 minutes they spent together. "At the end of that time, we were both smiling. That was the real treasure of being a volunteer. And she got 30 minutes not to think of her illness. She just taught me so much about the rewards of being kind, and I still think of her all this time later."

At times, hospital employees see a need outside the realm of health care that they can meet.

That was true in in the early 1990s, when several staff members in a unit that treated diabetic patients joined together to help a young mother and her son. Paula Rice, an administrative assistant, vividly remembered that morning. A 30-year-old man with diabetes was dressing himself before being discharged so he could tell his son he had to get his leg amputated, Rice said.

"This fellow was jovial and laughing and full of life. He was just a young guy with a 10-year-old son and a wife," she said. "He was a severe diabetic. The doctor had told him they just couldn't save his leg. The man said he had to go home and tell his son this."

Rice said she was bathing a person in another room when she heard a noise. "He (diabetic man) fell to the floor and died. He was putting his pants on to go home. He coded. There was no saving him. He was given CPR," she said. "We did all we could to save him but it was impossible.

"We were all stunned and saddened," she said.

The social worker at the time knew the family was destitute, Rice added. "This was a loving family who was considerate of others. They identified the man as an (organ) donor and wished that we would follow those wishes. Since there were unique circumstances in this tragedy, our supervisors put together a plan to help everyone involved."

They knew the family didn't have enough money for a funeral, so they decided to put one together at the hospital the next day. A nearby wing was closed and under construction, so one patient room was turned into a "mini funeral parlor," Rice said.

"We gathered flowers from some of our other patients and bought some from the gift shop, too. The staff that morning made the patient presentable for his funeral, and the hospital chaplain presided," she said, adding that the room had to be cool to preserve his body for organ donation.

About 12 people, everyone in the unit who didn't have to work on the floor, attended the service. "We all took a collection for his cremation and made the arrangements. The family was very thankful for his tribute. The room was beautiful," Rice recalled. "It was perfect.

"It shows how people cared for their patients' well-being. It is what epitomizes Bloomington Hospital," she said. "It is a moment that made us feel good about us. That's not something people do every day.

"Time passes and buildings age," Rice said. "What goes on in these structures are memories that the community and our IU Health Bloomington staff will remember long past it's time. Many dear ones have come into the world here and many have passed on."

One of the single events some hospital employees cite as memorable is the "Bud Kohr blind walk." During Kohr's tenure as president and CEO of Bloomington Hospital from 1966 to 1995, he had all new employees attend an orientation session on their first day to drive home a lesson he wanted them to always remember as they worked with patients.

It worked, said Susie J. Braun, a hospital cytotechnologist, who studies cells. She went through the orientation and walk on her first day in October 1992.

"Bud wanted us to know what it was like as the patient and the patient's family to be in an unknown situation. "I try, in my interaction with patients, to always keep that in mind. They are coming into something and somewhere that is unknown, and the unknown is always scarier than the known."

Unless you've walked blindfolded before, staff member Rice recalled, it's not possible to understand how hard it is to walk without seeing, while navigating around lots of obstacles, especially somewhere you haven't been before.

"It really was a very eye-opening experience," said Rice, a 31-year employee of IU Health Bloomington Hospital. She was describing the well-known "Bud Kohr blind walk" she experienced back in October 1989 during a new employee orientation session.

At first, she and about 30 other new employees didn't have any idea what they were about to experience. They were in the basement of the Medical Arts Building, which was being renovated, behind the hospital. Saw horses, eight-foot pieces of lumber, pipes, saws, and other equipment were strewn around the room.

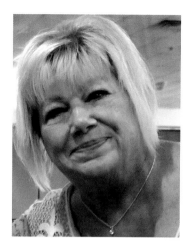

Paula Rice, a 31-year staff member at IU Health Bloomington Hospital, has served as an assistant in the behavioral health unit for the last 20 years. *Photo submitted by Paula Rice.*

Kohr started this unique tradition early in his tenure. It became a ritual that many people remember years afterward.

"He came in and gave a little spiel and told us we are all welcome," remembered Rice, now 70, who has served as an assistant in the behavioral health unit for the last 20 years. "He was kind of a people person. He walked the hospital halls frequently and remembered people's names. He stopped to talk to people," she said of Kohr, who died in 2015.

"Bud's up there in the front of the room and he's telling us what we're going to do. We didn't know anyone who we were in orientation with. He asked us to buddy up with someone in the room, and he told us we were going to participate in the Kohr walk."

The new employees didn't know they were about to do on this walk.

But Kohr first gave them some perspective, Rice recalled. "He said that people come to Bloomington Hospital to heal, and they are here in a great time of need—to mend wounds or say good-bye to loved ones. He said they're putting their trust in us to be compassionate and care for their loved ones."

Each team picked an "A" person and a "B" person. The "B" people put on blindfolds. The "A" people, including Rice, held onto the hands of their partners. Kohr led the pairs for about 15 minutes around sawhorses and equipment and up a stairwell and outside, and then back down the stairwell and into the orientation room.

During the walk, Rice said, she had to talk to her teammate and show her she could trust Rice. "It made me think I'm caring for that person. I've got to keep the person safe. It is a responsibility to lead them, not push or shove them. You don't want them to feel like they've lost abilities they still have.

"You realize, oh, I really need to be specific. I really need to hold on tight and need to be careful and make sure that person doesn't get hurt," she said.

Rice remembered when she wore the blindfold, she had to trust her partner. She said she thought to herself, "You don't want to make a fool of yourself and trip."

The whole experience was "a light-bulb moment" for her.

"When we got back to the orientation room, Mr. Kohr didn't have to say much because it was quite clear what the message was—that we must take care to lead our patients into the unknown and build a trust with someone they have never met."

She said the Kohr walk made her think about how important it is for patients to trust the staff, for staff to be specific about what they want patients to do and to reassure them.

"You came away realizing we were the patients. We were acting in those roles—putting our full trust in that other person," Rice stressed. "He wanted us to see how reliant people are on us. He wanted us to realize the responsibility we all had to patients.

"It definitely made an impression on me."

CATHY EADS: "WHATEVER I COULD DO TO HELP, I WAS ALL IN"

Practicing injections in an orange sometimes just isn't good enough.

Cathy L. Eads, an IU Health Bloomington Hospital nurse, said she was working with a terminally ill cancer patient in the late 1980s who was going home with intramuscular injections of morphine for pain. This technique is used to deliver medication deep into the muscles, allowing the medication to be quickly absorbed into the bloodstream.

She was a young woman in her late 20s or early 30s and had been a patient for several weeks on the oncology unit, where Eads had worked for 26 years of her career. "Before she could go home, though, we had to teach her mother to give the injections. That made the daughter anxious and the parents, as well, because they hadn't done this before," said Eads, who started working at the hospital in 1977.

At that time, patients and family members often practiced giving injections in an orange to simulate injections into a person's skin. Eads said this was before the technology of pain pumps programmed with intervals of pain medication available by pushing a button.

"We ordered an orange and did it. I started showing them. The daughter didn't think her mom could practice on an orange and then give the shot to her. It has kind of the same feel. But there was a lot of anxiety there," remembered Eads.

"The panic started in with her. She asked, 'Who is going to give me the shots?' She did not want to die there at the hospital. Somehow we had to make it happen because we wanted her to go home," Eads said.

"I never had been afraid of needles. My coworkers thought I was crazy," Eads remembered. "This poor girl, she had enough anxiety and stress going on with her. Whatever I could do to help, I was all in.

"I didn't want to put more on the patient. I wanted to reduce the stress. I then asked if she would like for her mother to give me the shot. So, when it was time to start giving them to their daughter, they would have more confidence in themselves, and most important, for the patient to be more at ease," said Eads, 63, who was born in Bloomington Hospital and grew up here.

"In most cases, everybody is okay with practicing on the orange. This young woman, bless her heart, she really didn't want them (parents) giving her shots. So the mother practiced on me with sterile water two or three times the first day," Eads said. "Then the next day, she'd practice it again."

The mother gave Eads shots in her arm and hip, and after the practice, the mother knew exactly where and how she needed to give the shots, Eads added.

"When the daughter was going to go home, the mother gave her daughter the shot. The daughter felt more comfortable about it then because she saw her mother give me the shots. The mother had more confidence, too."

When it was time for the patient to be discharged, Eads said, "I felt that they were ready to take care of their daughter at home, which made me feel very happy that I was able to help make this happen. . . . If this could make a difference for them, that was my thank-you. They couldn't thank me enough. Knowing that things were better, that's all I need."

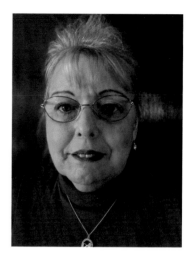

Cathy Eads, a registered nurse started working at Bloomington Hospital in 1977, worked on the oncology unit for 26 years and has been offering nursing care to people in their homes for IU Health Bloomington Home Care since 2011. *Photo submitted by Cathy Eads.*

"The patient was very happy that she was getting to go home with her family," she said. "She may have lived six more months."

Over the years, Eads has worked in several different areas in the hospital and worked with many patients. Many survived. Some did not.

For a short period, she worked in the intensive care unit in the evenings and then moved to the day shift on the medical surgery floor for more than seven years. In the mid-1980s, she started in oncology unit. Eads, who lives just outside of Bloomington in Monroe County, has worked for the IU Health Bloomington Home Care since 2011, giving nursing care to people in their homes.

"It was tough at times," Eads recognized. "It sure was."

When she was working on the oncology unit, some patients would come back every three or four weeks for treatments and nurses would often keep the same patients. "They became like family to us. We would see them quite often, so we got to know them. Continuity of care, that is extremely important.

"The times seeing the patients who got better and got to home—that was a really good feeling to see them and know that we made a difference for them. Those who didn't make it—that was hard. It was hard, but we did everything to make it as best as we could for them."

Some former patients come back to see their nurses. "Patients would tell us how they are doing and tell us they appreciated the care we got there. Patients would bring us a treat and something to show us their gratitude.

"Them coming back to see us—it would just warm our hearts."

PAMELA HODGES: "THIS BEGAN MY PASSION OF ENCOURAGING HEALTHIER MOMS AND BABIES THROUGH LACTATION ASSISTANCE."

For many years, registered nurse Pamela Hodges had a mission—a passion—while working as a registered nurse at Bloomington Hospital beginning in January 1981.

She was concerned that new mothers weren't getting the good guidance about the importance of breast-feeding for the health of their babies. At that time, she recalled, breast-feeding wasn't well

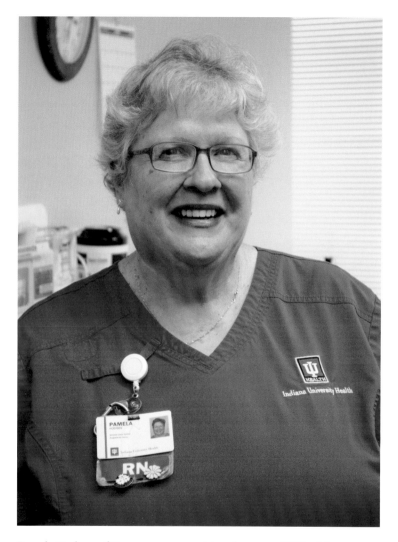

Pamela Hodges, of Paragon, now a registered nurse at IU Health Wound Healing Center, started at Bloomington Hospital in 1981 and worked primarily with new mothers and babies, focusing on providing lactation assistance as a certified lactation consultant. *Photo credit: Travis Tate, IU Health Media Services.*

accepted or encouraged. Many doctors didn't know much about it, she said. It wasn't the norm.

Hodges wanted to change all that. And she was one of a few people at the hospital who were instrumental in making breast-feeding more acceptable and practiced by more women.

As a new nurse working in the Special Care Nursery on the night shift, she spent a lot of time helping moms and their new babies during the first few days after delivery. She said another registered nurse gave a mini in-service class on the benefits of breast-feeding.

"This began my passion of encouraging healthier moms and babies through lactation assistance," said Hodges, now 67, of Paragon. In 1990, she became one of only a few International Board Certified Lactation Consultants in the state.

"The lactation program (at the hospital) began and was an uphill battle for many years trying to educate doctors and nurses on the benefits of nursing," she said. "Now, many years later, it is thriving."

When she first started at the hospital 40 years ago as a new graduate, she started working with women who had some difficulty with breast-feeding but struggled to figure out how to best help them. Another nurse went to a conference on the topic and shared her knowledge. Hodges said she also went to many conferences to learn more on her own, paying for her own expenses.

For example, she recalled on the night shift babies went out to their mothers only at 2 a.m. and 6 a.m., and the nurses would have to ask some mothers to put out their cigarettes. Nurses often gave babies glucose water because they were jaundiced and, unfortunately, that filled them up so they didn't want to nurse, explained

Hodges. "That baby will tell the breast how much it needed and when it needed milk."

Changing the engrained misconceptions about breast-feeding held by many health care providers and even mothers was a challenge.

"The nurses caught on pretty well, but it was pretty hard. . . . There were some old-time nurses who didn't breast-feed and didn't encourage it," she remembered. "It's a sensitive issue. It wasn't accepted at that time."

Some of the underlying reasons were that some women weren't comfortable with their own bodies, due to assault or other reasons, and breasts were looked at as sexual objects, she explained. "You didn't see women breast-feeding in public."

Most physicians who were ob-gyns didn't have lactation consultants in their offices because they weren't heard of at that time, Hodges said. In 1991, just a few consultants had passed their tests, which required 2,000 hours of work. "After I became certified, I felt like I had a lot more behind me. I did in-service at Ivy Tech (Community College) and went to doctors' offices. You had to keep it at the forefront."

She added that she became known as a resource person in the community, and the hospital started paying for her certification as a lactation consultant and her conference fees. "I had learned how important breast milk was for babies and how difficult it was for women to get to the point that they are confident in breast-feeding."

The issue surrounding the use of baby formula was also a problem.

"Way back then, formula was a real big thing," she said. Formula companies would court the physicians and encourage them to use their products, according to Hodges. "It was such an easy thing for the doctors to order. Even if their mothers were trying to breast-feed, they weren't sure their milk was going to come in."

Hodges also pushed against the long-time practice of giving away free baby formula to new mothers in the hospital, with the support of nurse administrator Dana Watters, who was director of obstetrics department at that time. The practice had to be dropped if the hospital was to earn the Baby-Friendly Hospital designation under an international program run by the World Health Organization and UNICEF. The designation was first accomplished in 2011.

"That was my fight," Hodges said. "I had a lot of support from a lot of people. Several obstetrics employees helped with that."

Hodges recalled meeting with representatives of the La Leche League and the Monroe County Public Health, who also shared their concerns with giving new mothers baby formula and sending them home with others products with the names of baby formula companies on them. So, they designed new information cards for mothers and did not include drinking cups with companies' names on them.

"We just kind of cleaned house and worked to change the mindset by changing what everybody saw and took home," she said.

While just a handful of certified lactation consultants existed, the movement was starting to evolve and a "snowball" effect started, said Hodges. "Dana (Watters) was just so supportive in getting everything started. We set up a pumping station at the hospital so (women) could pump while they were at work, too."

Once she was certified, Hodges said, she started doing educational classes for students and doctors. "I was kind of put in that role of educator when I was working in special care nursery. Pediatrics would call me. If they had a baby in trouble, I could come and help out."

The hospital's lactation program started in 1990 and started taking more of her time as she saw patients on an outpatient basis to help with breast-feeding and made rounds to help mothers of newborn babies, Hodges said.

"It's really important to have everybody on board to get the baby to the breast," she stressed. "It's important for their health."

In 2002, Hodges decided to make a turn in her nursing career by going to the IU Health Wound Healing Center, at 2920 S. McIntire Drive. The outpatient clinic has a team of clinicians, including nurses, physical therapists, certified wound specialists, diabetic educators, and physicians from multiple specialties. They treat diabetic wounds, surgical wounds, knife and gunshot wounds, and other types of wounds.

"It's been a wonderful ride at Bloomington Hospital," she said. "It was very emotional to leave. I loved what I did there, but I realized this was an opportunity that I needed to take. But it's been fascinating out here because it's been a whole new world. How challenging and exciting it is every day."

STROKE SURVIVOR FRED DUNN: "THIS IS A MARVELOUS SUPPORT PROGRAM. IT TAKES AWAY THE FEAR"

Fred Dunn, at age 65, didn't have any major health issues or heart problems. The Bloomington native and former U.S. Army officer was still working for an industrial supplies and manufacturing business.

Little did Dunn know what was about to hit him while he talked on the phone in 2008 with a business associate in Chicago.

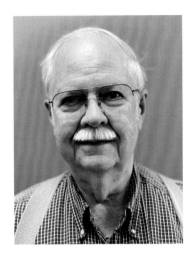

Fred Dunn, of Bloomington, suffered stroke in 2008 and was successfully treated at IU Health Bloomington Hospital. *Photo submitted by Fred Dunn.*

On the day of Dunn's stroke, he was calmly discussing a business matter on the phone when he suddenly dropped the phone. Dunn, now 77, said his associate realized something was wrong and got in touch with Dunn's sister-in-law, Susan Dunn. She called her husband, Dr. Allen W. Dunn, an anesthesiologist at the hospital. Dunn's brother came over and took him to the hospital.

"I knew something was wrong. My speech was slurred. But part of that time is blurry," he recalled. "Things change quickly. You don't really understand it until it hits you. You lose control and somebody else has to notice it."

Dunn praised the reaction of the medical staff. "They did an outstanding job. They started the stroke protocol of determining what it was and stopping whatever was happening. It was a real full-blown stroke."

But he said it's important to get to the hospital within about three hours of symptoms starting, get a CAT scan and the medication injected that helps prevent damage. Hospitals can administer alteplase, a clot-busting drug, if administered soon enough. The drug breaks up the blood clot and restores blood to the brain, eliminating or lessening the severity of consequences.

"I had loss of coordination on the left side, affecting my arm and leg. I had limited speech and a little bit of aphasia," he said. Aphasia, most often caused by strokes on the left side of the brain, is a language disorder that affects the ability to communicate.

Dunn said he was in the hospital about five days. His health team was concerned about him having a second stroke. Also, he said he was in a wheelchair for a few days and had physical therapy to help him get back on his feet and restore his balance and coordination. After being released, he said he had outpatient therapy for a couple months with very good therapists.

"I couldn't drive at first and had to work hard to get back functioning like I used to. They (therapists) knew what to do," Dunn said. "They were very professional."

Even now, he says speaking can be hard. "Sometimes the word you want doesn't come. A person's name may not come to you right away. I used to do a lot of public speaking, but I don't do that anymore."

He compared having a stroke to a computer breakdown. "Your computer goes down and you have to reboot your data. Your body learns how to get the same thing done in a different way."

Dunn said the hospital's Stroke Support Group has been a significant help to him. About 25 stroke survivors, and sometimes spouses, attend the monthly meetings at the Sherwood Oaks Christian Church. Speakers, including a pharmacist, dietitian, and city administrators, speak at meetings about medicines and side effects, good diets, local services, and other topics. He said he walks more now and has improved his diet.

"We talk about strokes, and what's going on, and the medicines. After you've had the event and gone through the rehabilitation, it's a time to sit back and say, 'What are we doing? Where are we?' And it's time to share stories with each other. The group members talk and learn from each other.

"It made all the difference to me. It's a whole new world. You don't know how it's going to affect you at first," said Dunn. "This is a marvelous program. It takes the fear away. Your whole world is falling apart and here's how you put it back together."

The free program, Dunn said, basically means the hospital is saying to survivors that it still is concerned about their recovery. "It says, 'We're here and still care about you.'"

STROKE SURVIVOR MIKE TILLEY: "EVERYBODY WAS AMAZED I WALKED OUT THAT QUICKLY."

Mike Tilley, of Bloomington, experienced the same level of quick, expert care after he had his stroke in mid-September in 2018 at age 69.

For some 10 years, Tilley had fibrillation, an irregular heartbeat. So, he was taking a blood thinner. That's supposed to regulate the heartbeat so one chamber doesn't beat out of sync with the rest of the heart, possibly causing blood to pool in one chamber and forming a clot that can travel to the brain.

"That's what happened to me," he said about his stroke. But he still was not expecting what hit him during the middle of the night.

He said he went to bed and got up about 2 a.m. to go to the restroom and fell down. "I knew something was wrong," Tilley said. "I was kind of semiconscious and on hands and knees. I could put my hand on the night stand, but my left side wasn't working. My wife said one side of my face was droopy and I wasn't

talking clearly. I said I'd go back to bed and will feel better in the morning. But she insisted I go to the emergency room. I was able to shuffle myself out to the car."

He said his wife, Carol, got him to the hospital in about 20 minutes. "I think she even ran a red light," he quipped.

Tilley remembered she pulled up to the emergency room and yelled he was having a stroke. "It was just instantly a couple of people came up with a wheelchair and helped me get into it. The first thing I know I was up on a bed, and they were asking me questions. Very, very quickly."

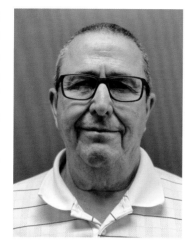

Mike Tilley, of Bloomington, suffered a stroke in mid-September 2018 and was treated at IU Health Bloomington Hospital and IU Health Methodist Hospital. *Photo submitted by Mike Tilley.*

A doctor asked him to hold his arms out straight, but his left arm was much lower than the right arm. The staff checked his strength and speaking and kept asking him if he felt where they touched him and understood what they told him.

"They knew right away I had a stroke, but just did that to determine the severity of it," said Tilley, who has been selling Medicare supplemental funds for about 35 years.

After a CAT scan, the doctor told him had an acute ischemic stroke due to a blockage of a major blood vessel going into his brain. Tilley said the doctor suspected a blood clot in the heart went to the brain, despite that he was taking a blood thinner. He had been taking the medication for about 10 years because of his fibrillation, caused when one chamber doesn't beat in sync with the rest of the heart, potentially leading to blood pooling in one chamber.

"They absolutely, absolutely did what they needed to do in not much more than two hours," said Tilley, now 72.

They recommended he be flown to IU Health Methodist Hospital by Lifeline helicopter because a doctor there could do a surgical thrombectomy, a type of surgery to remove a blood clot from inside an artery or vein.

After he got there, Tilley remembered the doctor said he could go in and clear the blockage by going up through his groin in a blood vessel, but there would be some risks, including paralysis or internal bleeding if the blockage breaks. "I thought I can lift my right arm and mumble and be understood. I thought I could live this way, if I had to," said Tilley.

"I choose not to do that," he added. "I prayed."

Neurologists and staff observed him every 30 minutes and his condition didn't worsen through Wednesday and Thursday, Tilley said. He said senior neurologists told him they don't see this type of good recovery very often from an acute stroke and that maybe it was due to him already being on blood thinner medication.

By 6 p.m. Thursday, the staff said he in good enough shape to leave. He said he had some loss of sensitivity in his left hand, but he could walk up and down the hall and stairs by himself. "Everybody was just amazed I walked out that quickly."

Within about a week, his left hand was better. Tilley said he gets tired a lot, but that was true before the stroke due to his irregular heartbeat. He also realizes he's more at risk for another stroke, yet he's glad that hasn't happened after more than two years. He said he tries to exercise and eat healthfully. He also enjoys going to the Stroke Support Group to hear the speakers, learn about new information, and share stories with other survivors.

"From the time my wife pulled my car up and by the time I got onto the helicopter, I could not hope for anything better. I've got nothing but good things to say about the whole IU network. I was almost back to normal within a month, maybe even a little less."

LAURA BALSMEYER: "I WAS JUST ONE PATIENT. IT STILL BAFFLES ME TO THIS DAY, THIS GROUP OF PEOPLE WHO WERE EXTRAORDINARY TO ME— THAT'S WHAT THEY WERE"

When someone with a major trauma or emergency arrives at IU Health Bloomington Hospital, health care providers react quickly as a team. Laura Balsmeyer discovered that soon after coming through the emergency room door. But she and her team didn't imagine how close they would become.

Laura's health—and life—changed significantly after she turned 40 in 2010. It's never been the same. Lengthy hospital stays, operations, incubation, sepsis, bowel problems, medications, and migraines all became part of her life. Health care providers in the intensive care unit played a major role in keeping her alive.

Laura and her husband, Brian, and her team agreed they all formed a special bond while fighting for her life. The Balsmeyers, formerly of Paoli, had an affectionate name for them.

"They were game-changers," said Brian, who coached the Paoli High School football team when her health problems emerged.

"They changed our life. Those people have a special place in our hearts. I'm really coming to tears now, that's how emotional it was," he said, choking up while recalling their care years ago.

The experience was quite memorable, too, for team member Raja Hanania, a pharmacotherapy specialist for critical care and diabetes at the hospital. "In 15 years in the ICU (intensive care unit), there are some situations which are unforgettable, and this was one of them. We all became so close to the family. They become part of your family. You don't count the hours."

Laura, now 50, arrived at the hospital in July 2012 in critical shape.

She said her health problems are complicated and the causes haven't always been clear. She now lives in Tuscaloosa County, Alabama, where Brian teaches and coaches high school football. The problems started with severe headaches and migraines about a decade ago, most often brought on by severe coughing.

She visited local hospitals, numerous clinics and had extended stays at migraine centers, including the Diamond Headache Clinic in Chicago. She said she took several medications that changed frequently to help ease the migraines but the side effects may have caused issues with her bowels, she said.

"I was trying too many different medications . . . There was something in there that destroyed part of my gut," she said. "But nobody has ever really determined that was why."

She got various diagnoses, including viral meningitis and pseudo tumors, but doctors couldn't really relieve her headaches, said Brian. He said her first hospitalization was in 2011, when she became septic and stayed at IU Health Methodist Hospital for 10 days. She was on life support and was given antibiotics to kill the infection.

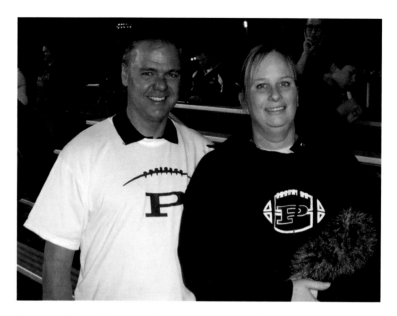

Laura and Brian Balsmeyer. Laura was treated at the IU Health Bloomington Hospital intensive care unit for about a month in 2012 for a serious intestinal problem and sepsis and later, a heart attack. She and her husband, Brian, formerly of Paoli, now live in Alabama. *Photo submitted by Brian Balsmeyer.*

Then in July 2012, she suddenly became unresponsive, for the most part, while at home in Paoli, said Brian. She was in septic shock again and had very low blood pressure. After going to Paoli Hospital's emergency room, she went by ambulance to IU Health Bloomington Hospital for what turned into almost a month-long stay. She was stabilized, but on life support, and tests found a serious problem with her bowels, Brian said.

The next day, part of her bowel was removed during emergency surgery by Dr. Bradley Ray, said Brian. The next morning

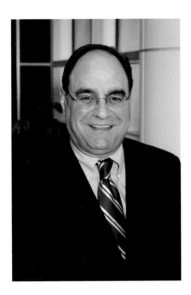

Raja Hanania, a pharmacotherapy specialist for critical care and diabetes at IU Health Bloomington Hospital, who was part of the intensive care unit team that treated patient Laura Balsmeyer. *Photo submitted by Raja Hanania.*

she took a turn for the worse and Ray told Brian another surgery would be needed to remove more of her large intestines due to infection.

"It was bleak and there wasn't much hope," Brian remembered.

Brian said he and their children agreed to the second surgery, although it was risky. Laura made it out of surgery, but doctors could not close her abdomen due to the fluids given to her to maintain her blood pressure, Brian said. She had an open wound the size of a small bowling ball.

Hanania remembered this time as a crucial period.

"She had very severe abdominal surgery, and her blood pressure went down very badly," he said. "There were 24 hours that were very critical. If she lost blood pressure, despite the maximum medication, she wouldn't survive. We were able to save her. She still stayed with us for two weeks after the surgery."

Laura doesn't remember much about this period until after she started to recover. But she recalled the kindness of ICU night nurse Terry Mason. "She helped me deal with a lot of irritation,

agitation and being scared and was very helpful with everything," Laura said. She also said her primary nurse, Cammy Felling, took wonderful care of her throughout her stay.

Another infection develops, though. Ray said he believed it would be best to move her to another hospital with more resources to take care of her wound and perform a skin graft over it, said Brian. Laura was transferred to the University of Louisville Hospital, where she recovered and her wound healed for two months.

Finally, she returned home.

The Balsmeyers were so grateful for the care she received in Bloomington that they wanted to do something special to recognize her health care team. Brian invited all 12 to the "senior night" home football game in September so they could participate in the coin toss to start the game and be recognized at half-time. Brian presented them with Paoli football shirts with "game-changer" on the back and had a hospitality tent for them, so friends and family could thank them.

"We wanted a way to say thank you and introduce the people who had been praying so much and let them see the team who kept me alive," said Laura. "It meant so much to me that they would take that time out of their schedule. We wanted to honor them throughout the town."

She said her health care team went above and beyond to help her and her family during a difficult time. "I was just one patient. It still baffles me to this day this group of people who were extraordinary—that's what they were."

Brian recognized the impact the team members had on his whole family and appreciated that they found a room for them to stay in sometimes, rather than the waiting room. "Those people have a special place in our heart. We thought we'd hit the lottery," he said.

Hanania said the evening also made an impact on the team. "It was very emotional. It put tears in my eyes. We were close when these things happened. We loved them so much that nobody hesitated to go down there," he said.

But her care at the hospital had another chapter—and her health struggles with headaches have continued.

She had more surgery to reconnect her bowel, so she could eliminate her feeding tube and eat normally. After all of that, she had a heart attack in August 2013 while she was home alone. Her family was worried about not hearing from her that evening and one of her daughters found her. Brian started CPR, a neighbor who was an emergency medical technician took over, and Laura was stabilized at Paoli Hospital.

But Brian knew where he wanted her to go.

"I planned her funeral many times over the course of the years. In 2012, the people in Bloomington loved her and so if this is to be her last days, I wanted her to be in Bloomington Hospital," he said he thought. "She's going to be around the people who love her—if this is the end," he said.

Fortunately, it wasn't.

Brian said she was put her in a medically induced coma in the ICU, and her body was cooled. The therapy worked. She survived.

The next evening, she was on the sidelines of his high school football game, he said. "We have so much respect and thankfulness that the good Lord put her in Bloomington Hospital."

Hanania said Laura was the one who refused to give up and fought hard to survive. "The bottom line is the patient. She was always doing the best she could and tried as hard as she could."

Under high-stress circumstances like hers, Hanania said, this case illustrates that health care has become more of a team effort than it was in the past. He said it's so important for all team members to work together, listen to each other, and communicate quickly. Multidisciplinary daily rounds are conducted every day on the ICU when they all discuss every patient in critical care, Hanania explained.

"Everyone on the team discusses all their (patients') needs and medications. The dietitian will discuss the diet. The physical therapist will discuss the movement," he stressed. "This patient would not have survived if we weren't working together."

He added that pharmacists' expertise is in medications, while he called physicians the best diagnosticians. "Doctors consult us all the time. We avoid a lot of adverse reactions. . . . Of course, we don't step on toes. We work with doctors. Now, we are part of a team."

He said, "A doctor told him once, 'If you think I'm the captain, you're the cocaptain.' This could not have happened, if we did not have this culture at Bloomington Hospital. There's no question in my mind that collaboration is the best way to treat patients.

"The bottom line," Hanania said, "is everybody is accepting of the fact that we have to work together."

Every hospital, every nurse, every physician have stories similar to these. The hospital's most important strength, as Rice remembers, is creating a culture where everyone can do their best and patients get the best care possible.

6

HOSPITAL STRIDES INTO THE FUTURE WITH STATE-OF-THE-ART REGIONAL ACADEMIC HEALTH CENTER

IF ONE TIME PERIOD in Bloomington Hospital's ever-changing and dynamic history could be chosen as the most pivotal, that era arguably would be from 2006 until 2021.

While other epochs were definitely significant, hospital leaders took bold steps in the last 15 years that will forever change the imprint and future path of the hospital in the coming decades.

In the eyes of many in health care and the broader community, the decision to integrate with IU Health and build the new $557 million Regional Academic Health Center places IU Health Bloomington Hospital in a much stronger position to adapt to modern health care advances and practices and better serve the needs of 467,600 people in its 11-county service region.

Health care leaders took the moves with much forethought and after struggling through considerable community debate over losing local control of the hospital and leaving the downtown area.

"I didn't go into it just thinking, 'Oh, we have to do this. This is a no-brainer,'" said Dan Peterson, board chairman of the IU Health South Central Region, about the vote to integrate with IU Health. "But I think everybody on the board at the time took it seriously and wanted to make sure we were doing the right thing because we weren't in a desperate situation, like other places.

"We gave it a lot of thought," he remembered. "It was very forward looking, and we were trying to be mindful of how the world was going to change around us and how we needed to be best prepared to work through that."

During the last 15 years, several key actions—and inactions—led the hospital down this path.

First, the hospital began purchasing land outside of the city in 2006, with the potential goal of moving its facilities from the land-locked site on west Second Street to a larger area suitable for a regional health care facility. The hospital bought 85 acres outside of Bloomington at Curry Pike and Indiana Route 45/46 for a potential new home in 2006.

Second, a 2008 task force developed four proposals to continue using its lifelong home on west Second Street. One plan renovated the existing facilities. Another was a phased redevelopment on the existing campus. Two others replaced the hospital to the east or to the west of the facility. Eventually, all were scraped for numerous reasons, primarily related to inadequate space and facilities, even if renovated.[1]

Third, the Local Council of Women, which created the hospital in 1905, approved changes in the nonprofit organization's bylaws in 2008 that allowed the hospital to integrate with Clarian Health Partners, now called IU Health. While the group didn't own the hospital any longer, its bylaws still gave the group some say-so over the hospital's 24-acre property.[2]

Fourth, after much public deliberation and some disapproval, the Bloomington Hospital board officially integrated with the

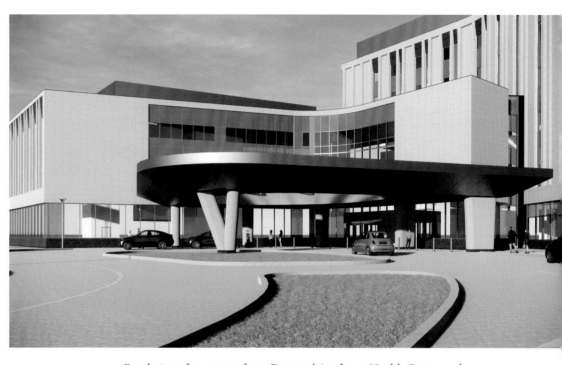

Rendering of entrance of new Regional Academic Health Center under construction in 2020 on the Indiana Route 45/46 bypass.
Photo credit: IU Health Bloomington Hospital.

sprawling IU Health system in 2010 and the facility officially became IU Health Bloomington Hospital. Merging with three other health care systems was considered, but dropped. The vote, in a word, was momentous for the hospital's future and emblematic of many small or independent hospitals' decisions to merge into larger systems.[3]

Fifth, a historic deal was forged in 2015 between the Indiana University administration and the IU Health system to develop

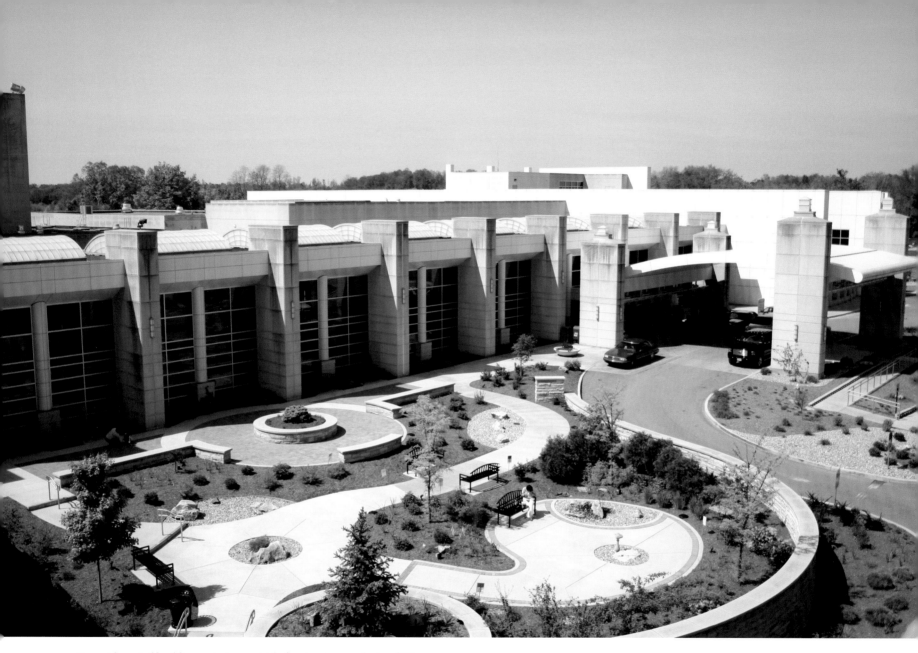

Recent hospital building exterior: outside front entrance photo of IU
Health Bloomington Hospital. *Photo credit: IU Health Bloomington Hospital.*

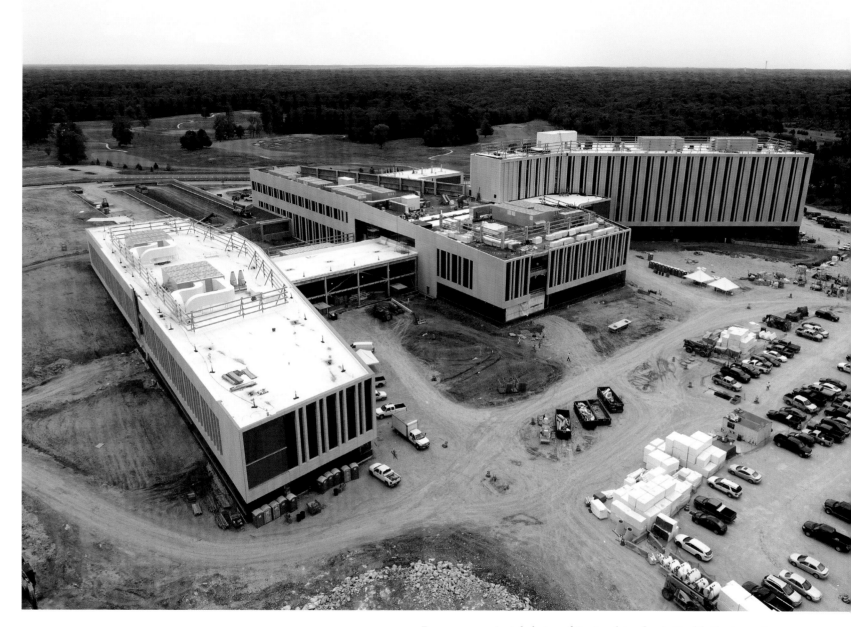

Pages 129–131: Aerial photos of Regional Academic Health Center under construction in 2020. *Photo credit: IU Health Bloomington Hospital.*

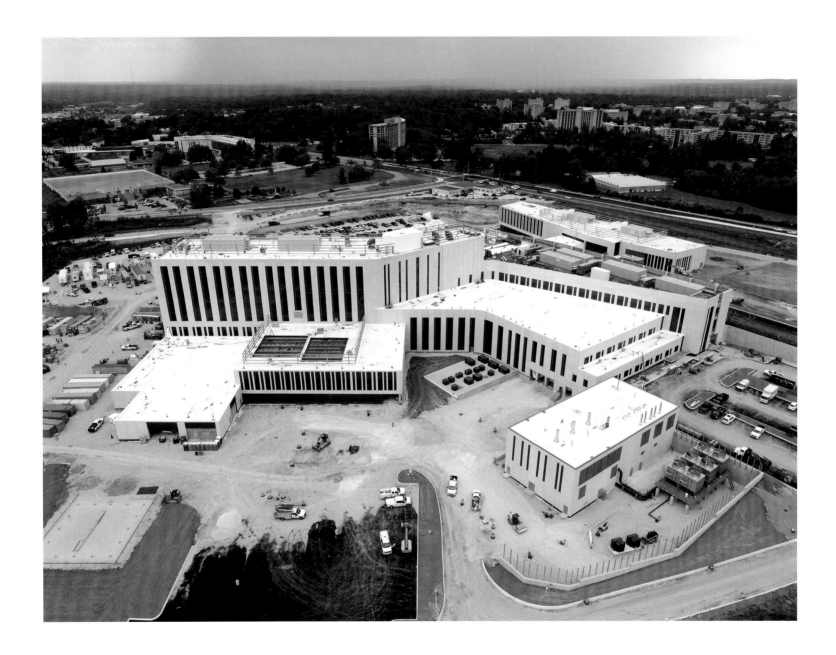

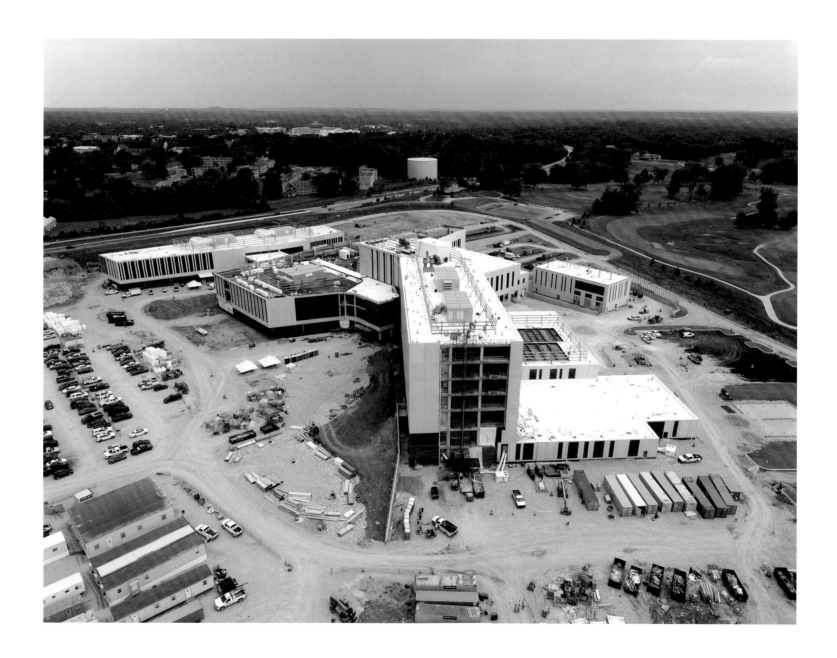

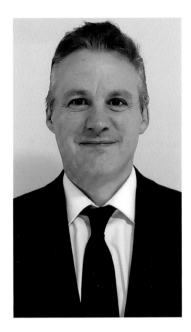

Ben Niehoff, current president of the Local Council of Women, is an attorney and co-owner of Slotegraaf Niehoff, PC, in Bloomington. *Photo submitted by Ben Niehoff.*

a new state-of-the-art regional health campus on Bloomington's eastside at the site of the former IU golf course. They agreed to build the IU Health Regional Academic Health Center on nearly 51 acres owned by IU off of the Indiana Route 45/46 bypass, combining the strengths of IU's academic health care muscle with the expertise and experience of the hospital's administration and staff.[4]

Substantial completion of the hospital is expected by late summer 2021, with patients moving in by the end of the year. The academic building was expected to be completed by the first quarter of 2021.

"It will be a major driver of community development, in terms of attracting people to the area," said Ben Niehoff, local attorney and current board president of the Local Council of Women.

"Having a top-flight hospital and academic center seems like it will do great things for the community," said Niehoff, the council's first male board president. "I think it would be hard to overestimate what that can do."

The fateful decision was reached after the hospital rejected using its current site—an idea backed by city officials and mayoral candidates—or moving to the west side land it had purchased for a new hospital.

Sixth, Mark Moore, CEO and president of IU Health Bloomington Hospital, stepped down in November 2016, after marshaling the integration effort and serving 14 years. The 15-month tenure followed of Matthew Bailey, former IU Health West Hospital president, who helped bring together the deal with the IU administration for the regional health center. Brian Shockney, initially hired as the hospital's chief operating officer in October 2015, was named CEO and president of the hospital and South Central Region in February 2018 on an interim basis and then permanently in July 2018 by the hospital board.[5]

Since then, Shockney has been guiding the development of the 620,000-square-foot hospital portion of the campus, which also includes an 115,000-square-foot IU Academic Health Sciences Building under the IU administration's direction. In the midst of that, Shockney and hospital health care providers have had to deal with the formidable challenges presented by the COVID-19 pandemic since early 2020.

All that has resulted in far-reaching change—even transformation—culminating when the new hospital and academic building open during 2021. But health care providers say the opening of the whole center actually will jumpstart a host of potential opportunities for collaboration between IU and the hospital.

Looking back, community and health care leaders recalled the steps leading to integration with IU Health as painstaking but ultimately rewarding.

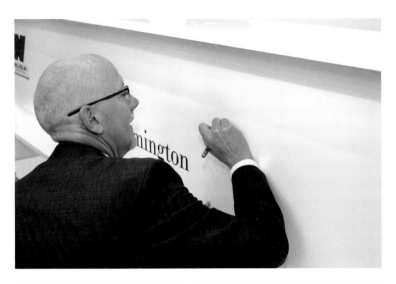

Left, Brian Shockney, president and CEO of IU Health South Central Region and IU Health Bloomington Hospital, signs a beam during construction of the Regional Academic Health Center in 2020 off of the Indiana Route 45/46 bypass.

Below, Brian Shockney (left, front), president and CEO of IU Health South Central Region and IU Health Bloomington Hospital, begins leading a tour of people looking at the construction site during 2020 of the Regional Academic Health Center off of the Indiana Route 45/46 bypass. *Photo submitted by IU Health Bloomington Hospital.*

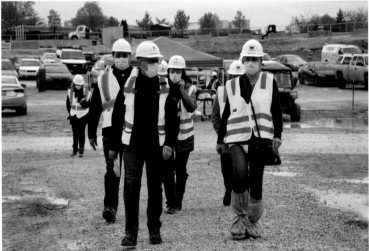

LOCAL COUNCIL OF WOMEN'S DECISION AND NEW ROLE

The Local Council of Women, a nonprofit group of local female leaders that opened the first 10-bed hospital in 1905, started letting go of its reins on the hospital in 1987.

That year, members decided to deed the hospital's west Second Street property to a nonprofit organization, Bloomington Hospital, Incorporated, which officially owned the hospital. The agreement stipulated, though, the hospital may not sell, lease, mortgage, or dispose of more than 5 percent of the property without the council's approval.

Then in 1993, the hospital board structure was revised and expanded to 18 from 12 members. The board included six members representing the council, six appointed by the Monroe County Board of Commissioners, plus an additional three members appointed by the medical staff and three by the hospital board.[6]

Three years later in 1996, the council expanded its own membership to include men.

But the biggest hurdle for the group came in 2008 after the hospital board of directors developed a nonbinding letter of intent regarding the terms of integrating Bloomington Hospital and Clarian Health (IU Health). Before they could proceed with finalizing the agreement, a majority of council members had to agree to change the bylaws to allow the transfer of land.

Not all of the members, though, were on board with this action, at least at first.

"This was a highly controversial change," wrote Susan Wier, who was Local Council of Women president at the time of the council's vote, in a written history of the council. "This was the most overwhelming period for the LCW board in decades."[7]

"Initially, there was a lot of skepticism and a lot of mistrust on the LCW," Wier, a council member since 2000, said in an interview. "I think mostly the basis of skepticism was having someone from Indianapolis deciding what was good for Bloomington and the surrounding area and understanding what are community health needs were."

Wier, a former nurse who owns an investment advisory business, First American Advisory LLC, added, "I remember distinctly how I was upset about it. . . . "I thought it would be an extremely difficult 'sale' to the community. And I didn't like that (Clarian) wasn't going to pay us for the hospital."

Eventually, most council members were convinced the integration made good sense. How?

"A lot, a lot, a lot, of meetings," said Wier. "We were meeting with hospital administration, with the hospital, board, and the people in charge of Clarian. The overriding, motivating factor for the hospital board and LCW board was to build a new hospital in Bloomington."

At one of those public meetings, according to a May 18, 2008, article in the *Bloomington Herald-Times*, hospital CEO Moore told the audience, "The status quo is not acceptable. We must either find ways to continue to grow and prosper, or we will move backward."

Wier recognized the time had come.

"Most of us feel our baby has grown up and it's time for us to let it move into adulthood on its own," she said at the meeting.[8]

Yet some members, including former council president Eleanor Rogers, didn't need convincing.

"I was one who believed it was the right thing from the get-go," said Rogers. She continued to serve as the council's representative on the hospital board until the local board was dissolved after the integration.

"I recognized the merger was needed because of modernization. It seemed to be if the hospital did not join with the Clarian people, the hospital would only remain at best a small community hospital and would have financial difficulties," explained Rogers, 80, former director of IU Health Bloomington Home Care. "It would have taken a long time to come up with the money to get the building needed and it would have been difficult to attract doctors."

Before the decision was made, Wier wrote, the council's membership grew from 110 to more than 1,200 in just a few weeks, as more people wanted to influence the outcome. "Both sides of the proposal were so hotly entrenched in their feelings that an armed security guard was posted at the voting meeting held (in June) at the Bloomington Convention Center. The vote was close, but the majority voted to merge," she wrote. However, that vote was contested and a petition called for a re-vote. At the second membership meeting in October, the vote again favored integrating with Clarian.

As part of the bylaw changes, the council retained its power to approve future bylaws changes for Bloomington Hospital and the right to appoint six of the hospital board members, including one each recommended by the hospital board and the county commissioners.[9]

With hindsight, Wier said she believes more positives will come from the decision, although that depends on how the mission is carried out by hospital system leaders. "We have to move forward. This is where we are and, and we're going to make the best damned hospital that this state has ever seen. . .You have to have faith that the people who are making decisions are making the best possible decisions as we move forward."

The Local Council of Women's role continued to evolve after the integration.

IU Health requested permission in January 2018 to dissolve the Bloomington Hospital board of directors and to form a South Central Region board consisting of community representatives from Bloomington, Bedford, Paoli, and Martinsville. The council membership approved the dissolution. The council was given one of the 14 seats on the regional board, as well as ex-officio position, and two positions on the nominating committee for future board members. In addition, the council now fills four seats on the newly created Community Health Committee, which received $250,000 from IU Health to advance community health initiatives, including tobacco cessation and infant mortality.

As part of that agreement, the Local Council of Women was given $500,000 to help promote community health projects. Niehoff, council president, said those funds were invested and the interest earned is used to support various efforts decided upon by the council's approximately 75 members. The council continues to meet quarterly for presentations from health care professionals about health topics and from a hospital representative to explain hospital initiatives.[10]

With those funds, the council has helped the Bloomington Health Foundation sponsor the Aunt Bertha Portal, an online portal that supplies information about community health care services, supported nonemergency medical transportation, and bought protective jackets for firefighters. Funds also are used to award college scholarships annually to students majoring in medical fields.

While the council has stepped back from running the hospital, Wier explained in the historical document, that members still are concerned about contributing to the community's overall health and well-being.

"It is apparent that change is consistent for LCW, and adjustments and developments as a result of the demands have been challenging," she wrote. "Today, the LCW remains the link between the community and the health care entity it helped to create, Bloomington Hospital. Combining tradition with innovative thought, LCW works with Bloomington Hospital to bring the best possible health care to our community."[11]

THE BIG STEP: PROS AND CONS OF INTEGRATING WITH IU HEALTH

Five months after the Local Council of Women's October 2008 vote allowing the Bloomington Hospital to proceed, the hospital board and administration began moving forward with an 18-month process to develop a regional strategic plan and facilities

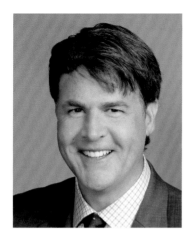

Jefferson Shreve, owner of Bloomington-based Storage Express, served on the Bloomington Hospital board of directors from 2005 to 2011, as the Local Council of Women's representative. *Photo submitted by Jefferson Shreve.*

plan that IU Health and the hospital board could approve.

But it wasn't until January 2010 when the board and IU Health ironed out all the details and voted to officially tie the knot.[12]

Before getting to that point, many community and health care leaders spent untold hours debating the pros and cons, evaluating finances, and figuring out the best and worst case scenarios of joining a larger, established health system.

For some, the decision was easier and boiled down to which system to join, not whether or not to do so. For others, the potential negative consequences loomed larger than others considered them to be.

To Jefferson Shreve, a hospital board member in 2010, it was clearly a milestone vote. The decision before the board initially was whether or not to remain independent or to integrate into a larger system, not which one.

"That was a major inflexion point in the life of our hospital system locally. That was the toughest decision," he said referring to votes during his two-term board tenure.

Then, the board determined pretty quickly the four options were Clarian (IU) Health, Ascension St. Vincent Hospital, St.

Francis Health Network, and Community Health Network, explained Shreve, owner of Bloomington-based Storage Express.

"When we were really wrestling with the decision whether to stay independent or integrate, it was the centennial of the hospital, we were strong financially. Our CEO was Mark Moore. He led the board through thoughtful consideration about whether we would integrate or stay independent," Shreve recalled.

Several members had attended conferences about the challenges of remaining independent, as health care was evolving and changing rapidly, he added. "Some, but not all, were of the mind that we needed to integrate. . . .The hospital leadership and executive committee had a number of conversations with the leadership of the four other networks," said Shreve.

The two Catholic-based systems carry with them a host of religious-based considerations that would be difficult to follow, so that's why they were ruled out, he said. Community Health wasn't as deep or large as Clarian, so it didn't take the board too long to settle on Clarian, Shreve added.

In the end, both Shreve and Peterson agreed the decision wasn't financially driven.

In fact, Shreve said integrating with Clarian wasn't the financially superior option because there was no exchange of funds. "Clarian didn't pay for Bloomington Hospital. We contributed the hospital into the Clarian system. We likely would have realized some monetary value with Community, for example. We could have engineered something like that, with some of the suitors we considered."

Shreve said the hospital agreed to deed the current hospital property to Clarian, but Clarian only committed to facilitate developing a replacement health care campus in Bloomington, without a contractual commitment, or agreeing to a time frame for building or an amount of money to be invested.

"We wanted to walk away with money in the account. But the board felt like Clarian was the best option from the standpoint of health care delivery in our home market," he stressed. "That integration, that pairing with Clarian, which had the most depth as a health care organization in central Indiana, and the promises made by their leadership, Dan Evans, the CEO at the time, and the CFO at the time, offered us the greatest long-term path to a promising future, in whatever form that took to move forward. We felt like they were the strongest system with the most breadth in central Indiana today and with the greatest commitment.

"They were hungry to add Bloomington to their base," Shreve added.

A year after the contract with Clarian Health Partners was completed, the system was rebranded as IU Health in January 2011. Clarian was created in 1997, with the merger of Methodist Hospital, Riley Hospital for Children, and Indiana University Hospital. Shreve said the rebranded didn't change the agreement and, in fact, the IU brand had greater value.

One of the driving forces, if not the biggest one, was the desire for a state-of-the-art facility because many agreed the current multiphased building wasn't structured well enough to adapt to evolving health care practices.

"We needed a new facility," said Dan Peterson, current chair of the IU Health South Central Region board. "There's no question that Bloomington Hospital was a strong community hospital. It was very difficult to provide best practice care in that old setting, in those old facilities. That's why a big part of the strategy going forward was to look at a replacement or revamped hospital."

Peterson, vice president of industry and government affairs for Cook Group, said the hospital was financially strong, and had good senior staff, board, and systems. Clearly, he added, health care was changing and the ability to stay financially viable was becoming harder with potentially reduced payments due to value-based care, coordinated care, and centralized health care delivery.

"So, the rationale of the board and the leadership, which was under Mark Moore at the time, was very much looking at the future," he explained. "A lot of hospitals were becoming part of bigger systems. That was a very typical thing and still is."

Merging with a larger system, Peterson emphasized, ensured access to funds at the lowest possible interest rate to build the hospital and access to tap into systems of best practices. But he said the hospital also was in a good position to retain strong independence and the ability to respond to local needs. "We spent a long time working through the details in negotiations with Clarian about maintaining enough local control," he recalled.

Having worked for Cook Group for 30 years, Peterson said he's seen the changes occurring in health care and understands the logic and value of integrating with a larger system. "We (Cook) have a lot of companies across the globe, and I was part of a lot of those changes across the years to help us become more of a coordinated, large entity of a system of companies. I saw the power of that, so that influenced me," he added.

But Peterson recognizes IU Health's expansion efforts haven't been perfect.

"The IU Health system admittedly has had to grow and learn how to be a system to take advantage of these opportunities," he said. "There have been a lot of stumbles not because the concept doesn't make sense, but you've got a lot of moving parts. They've tried to integrate a lot of independent facilities over a relatively short period of time."

Once all IU Health's new facilities came together, Peterson said, IU Health officials "were trying to honor local control, so they didn't force and put as much attention on everybody having to come together and do things in a coordinated fashion. That allowed everybody to get more comfortable with being a part of the system in the early part. But it also made it harder to change once you did start to be more aggressive and try to take advantage of being a more coordinated system."

He said some of that just needs to be worked through and the proper personnel needs to be in place. "So, you have to get the right people on the bus and the right people in the right seats on the bus," he said. "I think now we're really seeing that with the team we've got. Brian Shockney and all of his leadership team, bar none, in my mind, are really, really good and they are starting to really click and do some great stuff."

Attorney Lynn Coyne, who was chairman of the Bloomington Hospital board when the integration occurred, agreed that nowadays independent hospitals struggle, especially small, rural ones that would be even worse off without special Medicare funding they receive.

"The dynamic is really too large," said Coyne, former president of the Bloomington Economic Development Corp. "You need to be part of a system to be efficient, to keep your costs under control, and to be effective in this health care economy."

Coyne, now a member of the IU Health South Central Region board, said the whole idea behind the integration was to enable a "higher level of care for the community. How do you deliver in this tough environment the very best medical care to this region? You can't do it alone."

Being part of a larger system, Coyne said, helps hospitals control costs by taking advantage of economies of scale and gives health care providers access to the latest equipment. In addition, larger systems can better handle "hugely complex" management practices and payment issues, he added.

"Health care economics is a very challenging environment," said Coyne. "It takes a high level of understanding, involvement, and connections to be able to function in that environment. That's what being part of a system gives you, as well as just simply delivering high-quality health care."

While he said he didn't have any reservations about approving the integration, he recognized some people in the medical community and local community worried about losing local control.

From her vantage point, Joyce Poling, a former member of the Local Council of Women board and the Monroe County Board of Commissioners, said she also knew some people were concerned about losing local control of the hospital and being part of a larger system based in Indianapolis.

"They worried about how the hospital would reflect our community," said Poling, who served on the IU Health Bloomington Hospital board after leaving the county commissioners. "But I was not uncomfortable with it. It was a step that was better for the entire community. I felt it was the right decision."

Since the integration, local people have continued to be involved and decisions made have not negatively impacted Bloomington, she explained.

Dr. Larry Rink, long-time Bloomington cardiologist now practicing with IU Health Southern Indiana Physicians, sees positive and negative results of the integration. "There was good and bad out of that because the culture changed a lot. . . . The board has changed. The local board has become less important in the structure of things."

He recognized the new facility was needed because the current one is outdated. But he said he's worried the new facility isn't big enough for all the medical departments, such as orthopedics, that need to be located there, and is concerned about the potential impact to the public of higher taxes and fees to pay for the center.

Still, he praised having the academic health center near the hospital and the potential benefits of more closely linking the IU School of Medicine and health science education to the hospital. "Academics and medicine are one thing. It's important for academic aspects of medicine not to be lost. I think tying this in together is really important. Teaching students how to be doctors is totally more than delivering health care."

He added, "Theoretically, having IU Health involved should be better for us. I'm not saying it will be, but it can be. I'm not giving up hope that it will be. They should have more financial resources."

THE CREATION OF THE REGIONAL
ACADEMIC HEALTH CENTER

The prospect of a new, modernized academic and health facility opening on the east side of Bloomington, as part of the IU campus, wasn't on the radar at first. Ultimately, the unique option satisfied IU Health, local hospital leaders, and, of course, the IU administration.

Shreve, who was on the hospital board from 2005 to 2011, said, "When we served, there was no talk of that. No one knew anything about that. We didn't talk about that during deliberations. The academic health piece was something that IU President (Michael) McRobbie and others agreed to do or commit to, as part of moving the campus out to the IU property on the Indiana Route 45/46 bypass."

When he served on the board, Shreve said, the west side site, called North Park, was acquired by and planned for a new hospital, but, in retrospect, it wasn't a good location.

Shreve and many others at IU and in the health care community remain pleased with the change in plans, as the Regional Academic Health Center nears completion.

"We will move from here to the latest and greatest," he said. "We will move out of an older facility that's been added to in phases over the years. It's carved up and not seamless. We'll be moving out of an inferior facility to a superior facility.

"That's all good," he stressed.

Shreve predicted a lot additional development will be going on along east 10th Street, too. "I think you'll see more physicians wanting to move there north of town. There will be more higher-end housing developed out there."

Poling, a past hospital board president who now is assistant to the chancellor for Community Engagement at Ivy Tech Community College, said the new facility has numerous benefits, as the health care community continues to see "big leaps in knowledge" about providing better care and making use of flexible health care settings.

"Most people feel the relationship with IU and the academic health center was the reason the hospital was placed there," she said. "Research conducted there can be to the benefit of the community, too."

Poling recognized, though, many people who have lived in Bloomington all their lives have a sentimental attachment to the hospital. "When community has the opportunity be in the new facility and see the wonderful rooms, they will like it. As they come to learn and visit the new facility, they will become attached to the hospital," Poling predicted.

Planning for the hospital has changed even after the IU South Central Region board started to envision the new facility.

"The design, reach, scope and approach to the new facility is very different than what we were thinking early in how we would get this done," said board chairman Peterson. He explained it's become clearer that so much more care is going to be delivered in a lower acuity setting, which requires a lower level of nursing care. "There will be more outpatient care and more bedside care at home. Technology has advanced that it will really enhance our ability to deliver care."

Without the integration with IU and the shared space at the new site, Peterson said, the hospital wouldn't be able to do collaborative training for doctors, nurses, and other health care staff, as well and take advantage of other connections to IU.

Looking from different perspectives, Dr. Jean Creek, a retired long-time internist and former IU School of Medicine clinical professor, has some bittersweet memories of the current hospital and a few qualms about the new facility.

"It puts the building on the IU campus, where it probably should be," said Creek, who directed the IU Medical Science Program for more than two decades. "But I think it's more than bricks and mortar. I think it's the people who work in the institution. If something gets too big, you lose the camaraderie."

He wistfully remembered a time when the hospital's whole medical staff could sit around one table at lunchtime. "It would be 10 or 15 of us, and we'd get more accomplished talking about different patients with each other helping out," he said. "You never see that anymore."

Yet he recognizes the current building was constructed in a piecemeal fashion over the years. "You can do better starting over, but in a time when we have an overcrowded world and cement is one of the biggest contributors of CO_2 (carbon dioxide) in the atmosphere, it bothers me that we have to build a whole new structure like that."

The total 735,000-square-foot facility brings together multiple medical specialties and outpatient services into one setting. It also provides an innovation-driven environment in which IU and IU Health can partner to teach future generations of health care providers.

The day the new campus was announced in January 2018, IU and IU Health officials spoke enthusiastically about the opportunities that lie ahead.

IU President McRobbie said, "This plan will lead to the creation of the most comprehensive academic health campus in the state outside of Indianapolis and will bring together most of the IU Bloomington health science programs, and possibly additional programs, into one place co-located with the new IU Health Bloomington Hospital."

McRobbie also said, according to a release from the Bloomington Economic Development Commission, "This will considerably expand the opportunities for health sciences education and research at IU Bloomington, for innovative new programs

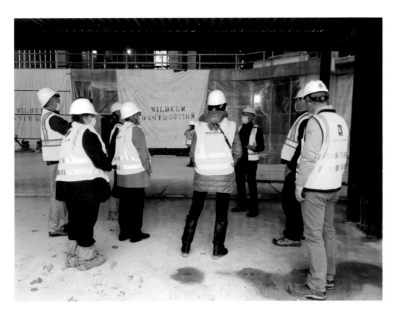

Brian Shockney (middle, facing forward), president and CEO of IU Health South Central Region and IU Health Bloomington Hospital, talks with a group of people touring the construction site during 2020 of the Regional Academic Health Center off of the Indiana Route 45/46 bypass. Photo submitted by IU Health Bloomington Hospital.

in inter-professional education, and for new clinical services at the new hospital."

He added the Regional Academic Health Center will bring together IU Health physicians, clinicians, and medical staff with IU faculty, staff, and students "in a way that will enhance and broaden the services the center provides and that will substantially expand the capacity for education and research by IU's health sciences programs by co-locating them in a dynamic and state-of-the-art clinical environment."

More specifically, McRobbie said the Academic Health Sciences Building will provide opportunities to grow IU Bloomington health sciences programs by increasing the number of students and, as a result, help to address the acute shortage of health care workers in Indiana. The release said he estimated the building, when completed, will house about 100 faculty and staff and train about 1,000 students.

Lauren Robel, executive vice president and provost at IU Bloomington, praised the center's future impact, too, in the commission's release. "The creation of a health education center next to IU Health Bloomington Hospital not only opens significant learning opportunities for our students, but will provide much-needed room for growth in a number of our programs. In many of these programs, such as nursing, social work, and dentistry, we could be serving more students than we do today, which eventually will be possible through this partnership."[13]

Attorney Coyne summarized the overall benefit of the center in stark terms.

"We have a half of a billion dollar regional academic health center being built in Bloomington," said Coyne. "You tell me how that would be possible otherwise. It would not have been possible. We would not be talking about a new hospital today, if it had not been possible to be a part of this."

THE FUTURE OF THE REGIONAL ACADEMIC HEALTH CENTER

Construction of the new medical campus is a collaborative project between IU Health and IU. IU Health is contributing $503 million to build the hospital, which is 80,000 square feet larger than the existing hospital, according to Shockney. IU is spending $54 million toward building the academic building, which will be home to the IU School of Nursing, and social work, medical science, and speech and hearing departments.

The campus will be a destination for healing, learning, fitness, and wellness, according to an IU press release. Among services and features of the center are:[14]

- Private patient rooms that will be much larger than most in the current hospital with ample space for family and friends.
- An academic building dedicated to the education of university students studying various health science disciplines.
- A variety of outpatient services, such as office visits with specialty care physicians and diagnostic testing.
- Inpatient services for intensive care, complex surgeries, and labor and delivery.
- A Women's Center for obstetrics, a neonatal intensive care nursery with private rooms, and other perinatal services.
- Outpatient or same day surgeries not requiring an overnight stay.
- A 24-bed surgical unit to serve mainly surgical patients who are in noncritical conditions and also sovme people admitted by the Emergency Department who need surgery.
- A hybrid operating room that basically combines services offered by interventional radiology, a catheterization lab, and a regular operating room. This will allow doctors to switch to an open procedure from a minimally invasive cardiac procedure after the operation has begun without transferring patients to a different operating suite.
- An Emergency Department triple in size compared to the current department, with 45 beds, including eight beds for behavioral health patients, which offers specialized care for conditions, such as strokes, heart attacks, or injuries to hands and limbs.
- A new Medical Observation Unit with 24 beds next to the Emergency Department for patients who need to be observed but not admitted.
- A trauma center to treat severe injuries resulting from incidents, such as automobile accidents, that entail multiple fractures, acute spine injuries, and brain injuries. With a trauma bay and other improvements, the center will be certified as a Level II trauma center with general surgeons, orthopedic surgeons, neurosurgeons, radiology, critical care docs, and other specialists available 24/7.
- A new proprietary app unique to the center allowing patients to sign any last-minute release forms and digitally perform many other pre-registration tasks.
- A simulated home with a bedroom, bathroom, and kitchen to allow emergency responders to simulate emergency situations and treatments. IU students will have access to medical simulation labs with lifelike robotic manikins at a simulation center triple the size of IU's current simulation facilities and which will be joined with IU Health's simulation center.
- 1,795 parking spaces for patients, visitors, students, faculty, and employees.

When talking of all the possibilities provided by the regional center, Coyne can't hide his excitement about improvements in the facilities and technology, as well as the enhanced partnerships with IU.

"Our doctors always had medical students that they've mentored and taught in their clinical duties. Now, the medical school itself will be part of the hospital. The nursing school will be part of the hospital," Coyne stressed. "We're talking about having residency programs. If we could get a family practice residency program when that hospital is open, we're going to be training family practice physicians here.

"That's huge. That's huge for Indiana, Bloomington, and the nation," he said.

He explained that residency programs are only operated at very high-level types of facilities to get the type of training needed with a large enough patient base.

"Now we have a regional patient base and the kind of sophisticated issues that residency demands. So, we'll be able to have a residency program. They're working on it now," he said. "There's a lot (to be done) from here to there, but we've got to get that hospital open and functioning. What residencies can we bring here? The IU School of Medicine is in charge of that. The facility has to be accredited for the School of Medicine to allow it to happen."

Coyne emphasized a residency program is just one of the advancements possible as a result of creating a regional academic health center, rather than just a regional hospital.

Significant changes and enlarging of surgery suites also will be a major improvement, he explained. "Now, the current hospital's surgical suites have fixed dimensions. It takes more space, the technology, and trained staff to deliver that level of sophisticated medical care. That's what the market demands out of you."

Simulators are used to train doctors and nurses, but that simulation center will be at the hospital, so the existing hospital staff will be able to use that technology, he added. "You have a complete, up-to-date simulation technology facility for training everybody. Plus, students have access to it.

"It's just really phenomenal," Coyne said.

Inpatient care rooms will be much bigger and more adaptable, according to Coyne. The total bed capacity in the center will be 364, eight more than in the current hospital. Of those, 198 are inpatient beds and 166 are outpatient or ambulatory beds.

"You can take an ordinary hospital room and turn it into an intensive care room bed. You have that capacity and flexibility, and you're not shoe-horned in and stepping over somebody else," he explained.

The hospital will follow the new course of medicine, he said, that "is not about putting people in the hospital, but keeping them out." People with complex, serious issues have to be cared for as inpatients, Coyne said, adding community health and population health will be stressed. "We've got to be treating people in their homes and in their communities to try to keep them out of the hospital."

He also is looking forward to seeing a "robust outpatient care facility," which will operate out of the center part of the hospital. "You can have arthroscopic surgery on your shoulder, and you don't spend a night in the hospital, unless something goes wrong. You have it, you get in our car and go home. That's the trend with all of these procedures," Coyne said.

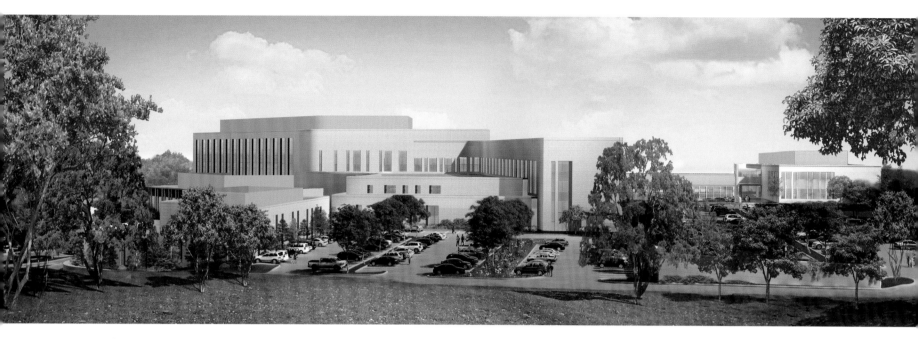

Artist's rendering of the IU Health Regional Academic Health Center under construction on property owned by IU on the Indiana Route 45/46 bypass. *Photo credit: IU Health Bloomington Hospital.*

The closer link to IU's medical expertise and facilities will have untold benefits.

"We're blessed to have the IU medical center nearby. This new facility will make our connection so much closer to the School of Medicine and medical center that all those great things that are happening are almost immediately available," he said. "We are so much closer to advances in genetic medicine, tailored drugs. We're so much closer to it now with this regional academic health center."

Dana Watters, retired executive director of the Regional Women and Children Center at IU Health Bloomington Hospital, said the new center "absolutely and unequivocally" offers so many advantages, as well as potential benefits due to the educational building on the campus.

She sees opportunities to increase the number of patients in the hospital who are between 20 and 45 years old, and that will particularly impact obstetrics. Watters said a high-quality and updated hospital in this great location can help to attract more businesses and people to the community who are in child-bearing years and women, in general, to live here.

"That's been what I'm interested in with the new hospital," she said.

Peterson echoed similar views by emphasizing the facility should not be considered a replacement community hospital, but a full-fledged regional hospital and academic health center. He pointed out that half of the hospital's inpatients are from outside of Monroe County, so the hospital's services need to be considered in that context.

ADVANCEMENTS IN TECHNOLOGY, PRACTICES TO BENEFIT ALL PATIENTS

The advanced technology offered and practices followed in the new hospital, Shockney said, will help better serve all patients and provide improved care in many ways. He foresees a variety of changes in health care delivery that the new hospital will be well-equipped to handle.

Over the next 15 years, he said, demand for hospital and health services will continue increasing with Baby Boomers aging. "This will continue to stress our ability to provide staff and resources to care for the population. We will be forced to invent new ways to care for patients without using people."

The new hospital has beds that weigh patients and place the weight in the medical records, he said. "Blood pressure monitors, oxygen monitors, surgical equipment will utilize AI (artificial intelligence) to make changes to the medication delivery, as well as care, based on the patient's vital signs. We already have AI for imaging that assists physicians in determining a diagnosis, given the thousands of electronic images one test can now produce.

Eventually, the diagnosis will be provided and only validation will be necessary," said Shockney.

He explained that physicians are no longer the primary care providers for patients. "Nurse practitioners and physicians' assistants are in high demand and can provide the care that the majority go to the outpatient physician for currently."

People will seek health care in new and innovative ways, Shockney envisioned. He said those ways include:

- Mobile apps, advice and tools online, urgent care, Fitbit and Garmin to tell cardiologists if patients exercised each day and how much.
- More wearable devices and implanted devices, and care delivered via diagnosis and treatment through text and pictures or video.
- Genome/genetics continuing to develop in a way that will either use genetics as a method for cures or to facilitate discovery of new ways for curing illness.

In the future, smart technology also will alert patients about the people who are entering their rooms and their credentials as they come in, Shockney explained. The technology also can reveal if the care providers utilized hand sanitizer as they entered or exited the rooms. "Apps will be provided that allow patients to register prior to their experience in any of our facilities, recognize them when they arrive, and guide them to the right location for their service," he said.

The landscape of health care providers will continue evolving and expanding, too.

"Nontraditional industries and organizations, such as Amazon, Walmart, CVS, Google, Apple, already have begun to provide health care and will continue to do so at a faster pace. They are developing technology to meet the needs of patients who will be utilizing the health system over the next 30 years," said Shockney. "The organizations realize there is a generation that will not adopt health care technology at a high rate, but they also realize that the future financial success is in building loyalty and connection to those who will be customers of health care from now until death."

Overall, Shockney said, patients will demand more efficient and effective care for a lower price.

"This demand will force health care providers to either transform or transition out. The new entrants will take the place of those that cannot transition quickly enough," he predicted. "We speak of concern regarding health care in rural and underserved areas. Once we have internet/web access to everyone in America, health care can be provided by anyone in the world from anywhere in the world."

With that in mind, health care and community leaders believe they are well-positioned to meet the upcoming challenges at the Regional Academic Health Center.

"It's another magnitude or quantum leap forward in health care for this region, much like that hospital in 1965 was," said Coyne. "There are hardly words to describe it. It's so impactful. People won't understand it until it's here or for a couple years afterwards.

"The folks who are working on this at IU Health have the vision," he stressed. "They understand it. The planning that's gone into this facility is just amazing."

Still, some people associated with the hospital for decades or who have worked their entire careers there have a slight pang of regret about leaving the facility and knowing it will be demolished. They also want to make sure the land is properly redeveloped.

"We've got 115 years of history, memories, and achievements here at Second and Rogers that there will be the sentimental regret over losing," said Shreve. "From an economic vitality standpoint, we need to be concerned about how the Second and Rogers site is redeveloped."

The city of Bloomington purchased the 24-acre property from IU Health for $6.5 million in 2018. The hospital system also has agreed to pay for demolishing several buildings on the site. But the parking garage will remain and perhaps the Kohr administration building, depending on further inspections, as of July 2020 plans. A master plan for redevelopment was scheduled to be completed by the end of 2020 by the Chicago-based architectural and planning firm Skidmore, Owings and Merrill, according to a June 18, 2020, article in the *Bloomington Herald-Times*.[15]

The city's Hospital Reuse Committee, a group of about 50 city officials and employees and local organization and business leaders, conducted the first of a series of four public-input sessions in June 2020 to discuss the future development of the hospital property. A cultural center, shopping opportunities, affordable housing, and a "mega-block" were presented as ideas to the committee, chaired by Mayor John Hamilton and former state senator Vi Simpson.[16]

"There will be a great economic development challenge as you hollow out that 24-acre campus," said Shreve. "There is a lot of privately owned property around there is occupied because of the medical-related businesses that will move out, too. They'll want to be near the hospital. . . . It will be a painful period of redevelopment of the campus over there."

Yet Peterson said he sees a great opportunity for what that site might be able to do in its next life for the community. "I think, to be honest, that has more potential impact when you combine it with the fact we're going to have this amazing new facility to deliver the really best care possible.

"That's the real exciting thing," said Peterson.

Dr. James L. Laughlin, a long-time pediatrician who serves as chief practice officer for IU Health Bloomington Hospital, has some mixed feelings. Ultimately, he knows the hospital will thrive.

"I'm sure there are aspects about (the current building) that I'll miss because I've been coming here my whole career, but I'm ready to move on," he said. "The physical plant isn't the important thing. It's the people and the mission that we're on that is most important.

"And that can continue in a better way."

NOTES

CHAPTER 1

1. IU Health Bloomington Hospital statistics on hospital usage for calendar year 2019, internal document.

CHAPTER 2

1. Bea Snoddy, historian for Bloomington Hospital and Local Council of Women, "Bloomington Hospital," manuscript accessed at Monroe County History Center, undated.

2. Bea Snoddy, historian for Bloomington Hospital and Local Council of Women, "Bloomington Hospital," manuscript accessed at Monroe County History Center, undated.

3. Bea Snoddy, historian for Bloomington Hospital and Local Council of Women, "Bloomington Hospital," manuscript accessed at Monroe County History Center, undated.

4. Bea Snoddy, historian for Bloomington Hospital and Local Council of Women, "Bloomington Hospital," manuscript accessed at Monroe County History Center, undated.

5. Pat Bartlett, "Argonaut Club program," written address accessed at Monroe County History Center, given April 1, 2003.

6. Cecilia Wahl, "History of Local Council of Women—The Beginning: 1897–1906," unpublished manuscript, 1995.

7. Members of Local Council of Women, "A Short History of Bloomington Hospital," brochure accessed at Monroe County Public Library, published Oct. 8, 1951.

8. Bea Snoddy, historian for Bloomington Hospital and Local Council of Women, "Bloomington Hospital," manuscript accessed at Monroe County History Center, undated.

9. Lee H. Ehman, "Women Step Up: Bloomington Hospital," Monroe County Historian, April/May 2019 issue, Monroe County History Center.

10. Cecilia Wahl, "The Women Behind the Local Council of Women," unpublished manuscript, Nov.14, 1989.

11. Bea Snoddy, historian for Bloomington Hospital and Local Council of Women, "Bloomington Hospital," manuscript accessed at Monroe County History Center, undated.

12. Bea Snoddy, historian for Bloomington Hospital and Local Council of Women, "Bloomington Hospital," manuscript accessed at Monroe County History Center, undated.

13. Members of Local Council of Women, "A Short History of Bloomington Hospital," brochure accessed at Monroe County Public Library, published Oct. 8, 1951.

14. Bea Snoddy, historian for Bloomington Hospital and Local Council of Women, "Bloomington Hospital," manuscript accessed at Monroe County History Center, undated.

15. Lee H. Ehman, "Women Step Up: Bloomington Hospital," Monroe County Historian, April/May 2019 issue, Monroe County History Center.

16. Bea Snoddy, historian for Bloomington Hospital and Local Council of Women, "Bloomington Hospital," manuscript accessed at Monroe County History Center, undated.

17. Lee H. Ehman, "Women Step Up: Bloomington Hospital," Monroe County Historian, April/May 2019 issue, Monroe County History Center.

18. Lee H. Ehman, "Women Step Up: Bloomington Hospital," Monroe County Historian, April/May 2019 issue, Monroe County History Center.

19. Cecilia Wahl, "The Women Behind the Local Council of Women," unpublished manuscript, Nov.14, 1989.

20. Members of Local Council of Women, "A Short History of Bloomington Hospital," brochure accessed at Monroe County Public Library, published Oct. 8, 1951.

21. Members of Local Council of Women, "A Short History of Bloomington Hospital," brochure accessed at Monroe County Public Library, published Oct. 8, 1951.

22. Bea Snoddy, historian for Bloomington Hospital and Local Council of Women, "Bloomington Hospital," manuscript accessed at Monroe County History Center, undated.

23. Members of Local Council of Women, "A Short History of Bloomington Hospital," brochure accessed at Monroe County Public Library, published Oct. 8, 1951.

24. Members of Local Council of Women, "A Short History of Bloomington Hospital," brochure accessed at Monroe County Public Library, published Oct. 8, 1951.

25. Bea Snoddy, historian for Bloomington Hospital and Local Council of Women, "Bloomington Hospital," manuscript accessed at Monroe County History Center, undated.

CHAPTER 3

1. "Hospital Drive Reaches Its 'Hour of Decision,'" *Bloomington Herald-Telephone* (no byline), Sept. 7, 1961.

2. "Hospital Drive Reaches Its 'Hour of Decision,'" *Bloomington Herald-Telephone* (no byline), Sept. 7, 1961.

3. "Hospital Drive Reaches Its 'Hour of Decision,'" *Bloomington Herald-Telephone* (no byline), Sept. 7, 1961; "$2.8 Million Hospital Drive Begins in 3 Weeks," *Bloomington Herald-Telephone* (no byline), Feb. 16, 1961; "Sarkes Tarzian Selected To Head Hospital Drive," *Bloomington Herald-Telephone* (no byline), Nov. 29, 1960.

4. Mrs. Leon (Jane) Wallace, editorial, "We Can Do The Best If We Have The Best," *Bloomington Herald-Telephone*, about 1964 (undated.)

5. Roland E. Kohr, "Building For Tomorrow, A message from the president," *Bloomington Sunday Herald-Times,* Dec. 27, 1992.

6. Pat Bartlett, "Argonaut Club program," written address given April 1, 2003, accessed at Monroe County History Center on June 30, 2020.

7. "Timeline—History and Events of 100 years of LCW and Bloomington Hospital," (no author) Local Council of Women, 1902–2002, unpublished manuscript accessed at Monroe County History Center.

8. Bea Snoddy, historian for Bloomington Hospital and Local Council of Women, "Bloomington Hospital," manuscript accessed at Monroe County History Center, undated.

9. William R. Baldwin, "Role of Monroe Community Hospital Association on Hospital Expansion," unpublished manuscript, undated.

10. Bea Snoddy, historian for Bloomington Hospital and Local Council of Women, "Bloomington Hospital," manuscript accessed at Monroe County History Center, undated.

11. William R. Baldwin, "Role of Monroe Community Hospital Association on Hospital Expansion," unpublished manuscript, undated.

12. Bea Snoddy, historian for Bloomington Hospital and Local Council of Women, "Bloomington Hospital," manuscript accessed at Monroe County History Center, undated.

13. "Calm Heads Are Needed To Solve Hospital Mess," (no byline), *Bloomington Herald-Telephone,* April 5, 1956.

14. "Hospital's Attorney Lauds Its Services," (no byline), *Bloomington Herald-Telephone*, April 5, 1956.

15. "$2.8 Million Hospital Drive Begins in 3 Weeks," *Bloomington Herald-Telephone* (no byline), Feb. 16, 1961.

16. Bea Snoddy, historian for Bloomington Hospital and Local Council of Women, "Bloomington Hospital," manuscript accessed at Monroe County History Center, undated.

17. "$2.8 Million Hospital Drive Begins in 3 Weeks," *Bloomington Herald-Telephone* (no byline), Feb. 16, 1961.

18. "Hospital Drive Reaches Its 'Hour of Decision,'" *Bloomington Herald-Telephone* (no byline), Sept. 7, 1961.

19. Bea Snoddy, historian for Bloomington Hospital and Local Council of Women, "Bloomington Hospital," manuscript accessed at Monroe County History Center, undated.

20. "Seventy years of progressive change," (no byline), Bloomington Hospital 1976 Report to the Community, *Bloomington Herald-Telephone*, Jan. 22, 1976.

21. "Here's What New Hospital Will Mean," (no byline), *Bloomington Herald-Telephone*, 1964 (no exact date).

22. "Seventy years of progressive change," (no byline), Bloomington Hospital 1976 Report to the Community, *Bloomington Herald-Telephone*, Jan. 22, 1976.

23. "For First Time In History, Hospital Prepares A Budget," (no byline), *Bloomington Herald-Telephone*, June 28, 1961.

24. Cecilia Wahl, "History of the Local Council of Women, 1950s–1980s," written in 1995.

25. "50 Years of Local Health Solutions," Bloomington Health Foundation, accessed June 10, 2020, www.bloomhf.org/our-work/#mission.

26. "Seventy years of progressive change," (no byline), Bloomington Hospital 1976 Report to the Community, *Bloomington Herald-Telephone*, Jan. 22, 1976.

27. Cecilia Wahl, "History of Local Council of Women—The Beginning: 1897–1906," unpublished manuscript, 1995.

28. Molly Cornbleet, "An Inspiration to Bloomington Hospital," *Bloomington Herald-Times* supplement marking hospital's centennial celebration, February, 2005.

29. Lauren Slavin, "IU Health Bloomington chief retiring," *Bloomington Herald-Times*, July 7, 2016.

30. "Seventy years of progressive change," (no byline), Bloomington Hospital 1976 Report to the Community, *Bloomington Herald-Telephone*, Jan. 22, 1976.

31. RATIO Architects, Inc., Indianapolis, *IU Health Bloomington Hospital Historic Resource Assessment*, February 2019.

32. Pat Bartlett, "Argonaut Club program," written address given April 1, 2003, accessed at Monroe County History Center on June 30, 2020.

33. Cecilia Wahl, "History of the Local Council of Women, 1950s–1980s," written in 1995.

34. "100 Years of Medical Excellence Remembered: A brief look at Bloomington Hospital's history," (no author), Bloomington Hospital publication, February, 2005.

35. Judy Talley, "Hospital fund drive expanding its focus," *Bloomington Herald-Times*, Jan. 31, 1993.

36. Roland E. Kohr, "Building For Tomorrow, A message from the president," *Bloomington Sunday Herald-Times*, Dec. 27, 1992.

37. Steven Higgs, "New era dawns at Bloomington Hospital," *Bloomington Herald-Times*, July 19, 1995.

38. Steven Higgs, "Independent hospitals face tough times," *Bloomington Herald-Times*, Dec. 14, 1995.

39. Steven Higgs, "New era dawns at Bloomington Hospital," *Bloomington Herald-Times*, July 19, 1995.

40. Steven Higgs, "Health Care at Crossroads," *Bloomington Sunday Herald-Times*, Jan. 21, 1966.

41. "100 Years of Medical Excellence Remembered: A brief look at Bloomington Hospital's history," (no author), Bloomington Hospital publication, February, 2005.

42. Steve Hinnefeld, "Bloomington Hospital to expand, renovate," *Bloomington Herald-Times*, Jan. 16, 1999.

43. Steve Hinnefeld, "Hospital renovation on schedule," *Bloomington Herald-Times*, May 23, 2001.

44. Steve Hinnefeld, "Hospital renovation on schedule," *Bloomington Herald-Times*, May 23, 2001.

45. Dann Denny, "Birthing center ready to deliver," *Bloomington Herald-Times*, Jan. 8, 2002.

46. Steve Hinnefeld, "Bloomington Hospital to cut employee hours," *Bloomington Herald-Times*, Oct. 9, 2001.

47. Steve Hinnefeld, "Hospital's president on way out," *Bloomington Herald-Times*, Nov. 15, 2001.

48. Dann Denny, "Bloomington Hospital CEO named," *Bloomington Herald-Times*, May 23, 2002.

49. "2004 Year in Review—Some Highlights," Bloomington Hospital News and Notes monthly newsletter, vol. V, issue 24, Dec. 16–31, 2002.

50. Emily Walsh, "A Large Celebration for a Large Contribution, Mark Moore Reflects on the Achievements of the Bloomington Hospital and Healthcare System," Bloomington Hospital release, late 2004.

51. James Boyd, "Hospital gala raises more than $85,000 for emergency services," *Bloomington Herald-Times*, Dec. 3, 2005.

52. Dann Denny, "Two hospitals ready to rumble," *Bloomington Herald-Times*, Dec. 23, 2005.

53. Inside IU Bloomington, "Kosali Simon named IU Bloomington's first associate vice provost for health sciences," Feb. 26,

2019, accessed July 10, 2020. https://news.iu.edu/stories/2019/02/iub/inside/26-news-roundup.html.

54. Inside IU Bloomington, "Kosali Simon named IU Bloomington's first associate vice provost for health sciences," Feb. 26, 2019, accessed July 10, 2020. https://news.iu.edu/stories/2019/02/iub/inside/26-news-roundup.html.

55. "Hill-Burton Free and Reduced-Cost Health Care," U.S. Government Health Resources and Services Administration, accessed July 5, 2020. https://www.hrsa.gov/get-health-care/affordable/hill-burton/index.html.

CHAPTER 4

1. IU Health 2018 Community Benefit Report, "Bloomington Hospital," p. 13, https://cdn.iuhealth.org/resources/IU-Health-2018-Community-Benefit-Report.pdf?mtime=20191112075325.

2. IU Health 2018 Community Benefit Report, "Bloomington Hospital," p. 13, https://cdn.iuhealth.org/resources/IU-Health-2018-Community-Benefit-Report.pdf?mtime=20191112075325.

3. "Fact Sheet," Bloomington Meals on Wheels, accessed July 10, 2020, http://bloomingtonmealsonwheels.org/factsheet.

4. "History," Bloomington Meals on Wheels, accessed July 10, 2020, http://bloomingtonmealsonwheels.org/ourhistory.

5. "Monroe County health rankings," Robert Wood Johnson Foundation County Health Rankings, Monroe, 2019, accessed July 15, 2020. https://www.countyhealthrankings.org/app/indiana/2019/rankings/monroe/county/outcomes/overall/snapshot.

6. "GOAL—Get On Board Active Living," IU Health Bloomington, accessed July 12, 2020, https://iuhealth.org/in-the-community/south-central-region/goal-get-onboard-active-living#.

7. "Performance Improvement," The Joint Commission on Accreditation of Healthcare Organization, accessed June 15, 2020, https://www.jointcommission.org/performance-improvement.

8. "Ten Steps to Successful Breastfeeding," Baby-Friendly Hospital Initiative launched by the World Health Organization and UNICEF, accessed July 14, 2020, www.tensteps.org.

9. "Primary Stroke Center Certification," The Joint Commission on Accreditation of Healthcare Organizations, accessed June 30, 2020, https://www.jointcommission.org/accreditation-and-certification/certification/certifications-by-setting/hospital-certifications/stroke-certification/advanced-stroke/primary-stroke-center/.

10. IU Health Bloomington Hospice House, IU Health, accessed July 24, 2020, https://iuhealth.org/find-locations/iu-health-bloomington-hospice-house-iu-health-bloomington-hospice-house-2810-s-deborah-dr.

11. "Hospice – Compassionate, Family-centered, end-of-life care," IU Health Hospice, accessed July 8, 2020, https://iuhealth.org/find-medical-services/hospice.

12. Joan Olcott, handwritten letter to Julie Darling, IU Health nurse navigator about donation to Olcott Center for Breast Health, 2018, accessed at Monroe County History Center.

13. Michelle Henderson, "Olcott Center for Breast Health helps cancer patients find sources of healing and strength," *Bloomington Herald-Times*, April 20, 1999.

14. Joan Olcott, handwritten letter to Julie Darling, IU Health nurse navigator about donation to Olcott Center for Breast Health, 2018, accessed at Monroe County History Center.

15. Michelle Henderson, "Olcott Center for Breast Health helps cancer patients find sources of healing and strength," *Bloomington Herald-Times*, April 20, 1999.

16. "50 years of local health solutions," Bloomington Health Foundation, accessed on July 1, 2020, www.bloomhf.org/our-work/.

17. Thomas J. Matzen v. US Department of Health and Human Services, 632 F. Supp. 785 (N.D. Ill. 1986), Memorandum Opinion and Order by District Judge Ilana Rovner, in Justia legal information website, April 4, 1986, accessed on July 16, 2020, https://law.justia.com/cases/federal/district-courts/FSupp/632/785/2260187/.

18. "Today Baby Doe Died," Down Syndrome Prenatal Testing, written by Mark Leach, accessed July 5, 2020, https://heinonline.org/HOL/LandingPage?handle=hein.journals/ilmed2&div=22&id=&page=.

19. Thomas J. Matzen v. US Department of Health and Human Services, 632 F. Supp. 785 (N.D. Ill. 1986), Memorandum Opinion and Order by District Judge Ilana Rovner, in Justia legal information website, April 4, 1986, accessed on July 16, 2020, https://law.justia.com/cases/federal/district-courts/FSupp/632/785/2260187/.

20. Jeff Lyon, "The Death of Baby Doe," *Chicago Tribune*, Feb. 10, 1985, https://www.chicagotribune.com/news/ct-xpm-1985-02-10-8501080761-story.html.

21. Gena Asher, "Out of the baby business—Retirement keeps this Bloomington physician busy," Feb. 17, 1992, https://www.hoosiertimes.com/herald_times_online/uncategorized/out-of-the-baby-business---retirement-keeps-this-bloomington-physician-busy/article_e30a4d32-ddbc-51a5-a9ea-23154b51d0b0.html.

22. Bruce Kappel, "Baby Does and the Right to Lifesaving Treatment," Minnesota Department of Administration, Council on Developmental Disabilities, Moral and Ethical Issues Specific to Developmental Disabilities: Guardianship, Involuntary Servitude, Sterilization, Baby Doe, Euthanasia, October 2009, https://mn.gov/mnddc/honoring-choices/cnnReports/Moral_and_Ethical_Issues4-Baby-Doe-Kappel.pdf.

23. Jack Resnik, "The Baby Doe Rules," report published by the Embryo Project Encyclopedia, May 12, 2011, https://embryo.asu.edu/pages/baby-doe-rules-1984.

24. Mark R. Mercurio, author, "The Aftermath of Baby Doe and Evolution of Newborn Intensive Care, Georgia State University Law Review, vol. 25, issue 4, Article 9, 2009.

CHAPTER 6

1. Rachel Bunn, "Final Stage: Accept it," with graphic, "IU Health Bloomington Hospital options for staying put," *Bloomington Herald-Times*, March 1, 2018.

2. Dann Denny, "Decision Time," with graphic, "Council's history," *Bloomington Herald-Times*, May 18, 2008.

3. Dann Denny, "Hospitals Seal Deal," *Bloomington Herald-Times*, Jan. 7, 2010.; Chris Fyall, "Merger is Clarian Health's latest step in building statewide entity," *Bloomington Herald-Times*, Jan. 7, 2010.

4. Michael Reschke, "Academic health center would give IU programs rooms to grow," *Bloomington Herald-Times*, April 16, 2015; Bloomington Economic Development Commission news release on IU, IU Health, and IU Health Bloomington Hospital announcing agreement to build new regional academic health center, accessed July 2, 2020, https://bloomingtonedc.com/iu-iu-health-bloomington-hospital-announce-new-health-complex/.

5. Lauren Slavin, "IU Health Bloomington chief retiring," *Bloomington Herald-Times*, July 7, 2016.

6. Dann Denny, "Decision Time," with graphic, "Council's history," *Bloomington Herald-Times*, May 18, 2008.

7. Susan Wier, former president of Local Council of Women, "My Monroe County story regarding the Local Council of Women," written council history used by the Monroe County Historical Society for series of articles for Monroe County bicentennial, March 22, 2020.

8. Dann Denny, "Decision Time," with graphic, "Council's history," *Bloomington Herald-Times*, May 18, 2008.

9. Susan Wier, former president of Local Council of Women, "My Monroe County story regarding the Local Council of Women," written council history used by the Monroe County Historical Society for series of articles for Monroe County bicentennial, March 22, 2020.

10. Susan Wier, former president of Local Council of Women, "My Monroe County story regarding the Local Council of Women," written council history used by the Monroe County Historical Society for series of articles for Monroe County bicentennial, March 22, 2020.

11. Susan Wier, former president of Local Council of Women, "My Monroe County story regarding the Local Council of Women," written council history used by the Monroe County Historical Society for series of articles for Monroe County bicentennial, March 22, 2020.

12. Dann Denny, "Hospitals Seal Deal," *Bloomington Herald-Times,* Jan. 7, 2010.

13. Bloomington Economic Development Commission news release on IU, IU Health, and IU Health Bloomington Hospital announcing agreement to build new regional academic health center, accessed July 2, 2020, https://bloomingtonedc.com/iu-iu-health-bloomington-hospital-announce-new-health-complex/.

14. Indiana University News Release, "IU Health, IU break ground on IU Health Regional Academic Center," Jan. 16, 2018.; Ernest Rollins, "Price tag for new hospital rises to $557 million," *Bloomington Herald-Times,* Sept. 24, 2019.; Dann Denny, "IU Health Bloomington Hospital adding staff, sharing expertise, technology," *Bloomington Herald-Times*, April 8, 2012.

15. Kurt Christian, "City to purchase current IU Health Bloomington Hospital downtown site," *Bloomington Herald-Times*, Jan. 3, 2018; Emily Ernsberger, "Series of public comment sessions on hospital site redevelopment kick off," *Bloomington Herald-Times*, June 18, 2020.

16. Emily Ernsberger, "Series of public comment sessions on hospital site redevelopment kick-off," *Bloomington Herald-Times*, June 18, 2020; Emily Ernsberger, "Green space designs proposed at second hospital site redevelopment session," *Bloomington Herald-Times,* Aug. 8, 2020.

BLOOMINGTON HOSPITAL TIMELINE AND NATIONAL HISTORIC EVENTS

Note: Years in black indicate national and international events.

1897 Representatives of local civic and philanthropic groups banded together to form the Local Council of Women, who wanted to address health and other community issues.

1904 Local railroad accident resulted in death of Lawrence Mitts, 32. Bloomington did not have a hospital facility to care for him and Local Council of Women members were moved to develop a facility.

1905 Local Council of Women organized and raised $8,500 to buy and repair a 10-room red brick farmhouse for the first Bloomington Hospital, formally dedicated in November 1905.

1918 End of World War I declared.

1918 New hospital was built and constructed with 35 beds. Old red brick building became the new nurses' home.

1920 Hospital admitted 78 patients, under leadership of Superintendent Harriet Jones. Discussion of X-ray machine started.

1923 Smallpox-scarlet fever epidemic struck country.

1928 Anna Nelson appointed hospital administrator by Local Council of Women and served until 1960.

1929 Penicillin discovered by Scottish bacteriologist Alexander Fleming.

1930 Great Depression hit country, leading to high unemployment and a large number of indigent patients. Serious diseases, such as polio, threatened public health.

1944 Hospital received federal grant of $92,000 and matching funds from a community campaign to support new hospital construction.

1945 Returning US veterans who fought in World War II increased need for hospital capacity.

1945 The hospital concluded its School of Practical Nursing, which began in 1906 to train nurses to serve in the hospital and resulted in graduating 124 nurses.

1947 Bloomington Hospital expansion completed, bringing the capacity to 75 beds and 25 bassinets and included a technologically advanced radiology department and state-of-the-art surgery rooms.

1951 Hospital pathology laboratory opened under direction of pathologist, Dr. Anthony "Tony" Pizzo, who led department 49 years and was known for professionalizing medical practices throughout hospital.

1954 Dr. Jonas Salk developed polio vaccine.

1956 Approval obtained from hospital board for a 147-bed addition costing $4.7 million.

1960 John H. Shephard appointed hospital administrator and resigned in 1966 to accept another position.

1961 Pink Ladies, the hospital's auxiliary organization, was created within hospital to provide volunteers and a source of monetary gifts.

1965 Hospital's 147-bed expansion was completed. New spaces were created for X-ray unit expansion, physical therapy area, and other improvements.

1965 Federal Medicare and Medicaid programs were created.

1965 Bloomington Hospital Foundation was created to raise funds for hospital programs and needs and was incorporated in 1967.

1966 Roland "Bud" Kohr was appointed president and CEO of Bloomington Hospital, retired in 1995, and died in 2015 at age 83.

1967 Hospital established one of the state's first cardiac intensive care units.

1970 Construction of $5.2 million expansion began in August and was completed in 1972, adding 159 beds and bringing total to about 300 beds. Total capacity included additional beds added on fourth and fifth floors, shelled-in during original construction of main building.

1971 Hospital establishes 24-hour emergency care

1972 Mental health clinic and Medical Education Department were established by hospital.

1981 Centers for Disease Control and Prevention and California Board of Health identify AIDS.

1981 Hospital began $24 million expansion and renovation project, which was finished in 1983, including new facilities for orthopedics, physical therapy, occupational therapy, surgery, critical care, and the 200-seat Wegmiller Auditorium.

1982 The birth of "Baby Doe," born with Down syndrome and a birth defect preventing him from eating, thrust Bloomington Hospital into national spotlight over parental rights to decide on lifesaving treatment for children born with disabilities. Baby died at six days old.

1985 Rebound Rehabilitation and Sports Medicine, a physical therapy facility, opened by hospital.

1987 A not-for-profit organization, Bloomington Hospital Incorporated, was created to assume ownership of the hospital from the Local Council of Women.

1987 Hospice of Bloomington became a hospital department, after first being formed in 1979 as a nonprofit community organization.

1988 Bloomington Hospital's Cook Cardiac Catheterization Laboratory opened, with major financial support from Gayle and Bill Cook, local billionaire entrepreneur who owned Cook Group.

1995 First nonviral whole genome sequenced.

1995 Nancy Carlstedt named president and CEO of hospital and left in 2002.

1995 Heart treatment advanced at Bloomington Hospital to include bypass surgery, angioplasty, and valve replacement.

1998 Promptcare East and West locations purchased by hospital.

1999 Hospital purchased Orange County Hospital and primary care practices in Mitchell and Ellettsville.

2000 Hospital approved and began $34 million expansion and renovation project, adding nearly 100,000 square feet of new space and renovating about 82,000 square feet to improve access to outpatient services and create a new obstetrics ward next to the pediatric ward.

2000 35 million people living with AIDS worldwide.

2002 Mark Moore named as president and CEO of hospital and retired in 2016.

2002 Larger neonatal intensive care unit opened in January 2002.

2004 Final renovation/expansion was completed, including a new, family-friendly birthing center, emergency room expansion, a redesigned atrium entrance, and some parking modifications.

2005 Bloomington Hospital celebrated its centennial anniversary. The Centennial Plaza, including the Charles "Pete" and Barbara Dunn Garden and Hospice Sanctuary, was dedicated.

2005 Bloomington Hospital's Regional Cancer Institute added high-tech, intensity-modulated radiation therapy and image-guided radiation therapy at its Radiation Oncology Centers.

2006 Hospital purchased 85 acres just outside of the city in the North Park tax increment financing district.

2007 Bloomington Hospital's Regional Cancer Institute received approval with commendation from the American College of Surgeons' Commission on Cancer, and earned the 2007 Commission on Cancer New Program Outstanding Achievement Award for its care for cancer patients.

2007 Bloomington Hospital achieved Primary Stroke Center certification and continues to renew that status every two years afterward.

2007 Bloomington Hospital announced it will begin exploring an integration with Clarian Health Partners.

2008 Local Council of Women voted in June and October to allow Bloomington Hospital to integrate with Clarian Health.

2008 A newly renovated unit on Bloomington Hospital's fourth floor was dedicated to caring for orthopedics and neuroscience patients.

2010 Hospital received "Magnet" designation from American Nurses Association for superior nursing services and practices. Honor renewed in 2014 and 2020.

2010 Bloomington Hospital officially integrated with Clarian Health, an Indiana-based, private nonprofit organization which combined Methodist Hospital, IU Hospital, and Riley Hospital for Children. Bloomington Hospital renamed IU Health Bloomington Hospital.

2011 Clarian Health changed its name to IU Health. Incumbent Mayor Mark Kruzan and challenger John Hamilton debate the potential physical move of the hospital during the primary election.

2015 IU Health Bloomington Hospital announced it is not feasible to stay in its downtown location.

2016 Matthew Bailey was appointed as president and CEO of hospital and left in early 2018 after 15 months.

2018 IU administration and IU Health broke ground for the new Regional Academic Health Center, on the Indiana Route 45/46 bypass at the site of the former IU golf course.

2018 City of Bloomington agreed to spend $6.5 million to purchase the current 24-acre IU Health Bloomington Hospital site. IU Health agreed to spend up to $8 million to demolish most of buildings.

2018 Brian Shockney named president and CEO of IU South Central Region and IU Health Bloomington Hospital on interim basis in February and on a permanent basis in July. Initially, he was the hospital's chief operating officer beginning in October 2015.

2019 IU Health officials estimated cost of the 735,000-square-foot Regional Academic Health Center to be $557 million, up from $400 million. IU Health's hospital portion was estimated at $503 million; IU's cost for Health Sciences building estimated at $54 million. Hospital's completion date was moved to late summer 2021; academic build completion date moved to first quarter of 2021.

2020 The city's Hospital Reuse Committee, a group of about 50 city, community and business leaders, conducted in June the first of four public sessions on redeveloping the hospital property.

2020 IU Health staff provide health care for COVID-19 patients beginning in March during international pandemic.

Information sources Bloomington Hospital Centennial Power-Point Presentation; *Bloomington Herald-Telephone* article, March 1, 2015, "Final stage of dealing with Bloomington Hospital's decision to move: Accept it"; IU Health Bloomington Hospital administration.

WITH HEARTFELT THANKS TO OUR COMMUNITY

Through the vision of leadership and caregivers, IU Health Bloomington Hospital has changed and improved to meet the needs of our community. We honor those who went before us, setting high standards for healthcare delivery. The realization of these ideals would not have been possible without philanthropic support.

Our heartfelt thanks go to all donors who contributed to IU Health Bloomington Hospital. Your support has been invaluable in advancing our mission.

All gifts are valuable to us. In this book, we acknowledge dedicated named spaces in IU Health Bloomington Hospital, endowed awards that provide financial or educational stipends to outstanding team members, and those who donated $10,000 or more to the Bloomington Hospital Foundation through 2017. In 2018, the IU Health Foundation became the philanthropic arm for IU Health. The IUH Foundation will recognize gifts made after January 1, 2018, to the Regional Academic Health Center at a later time.

DONORS

John and Patty Abshire
Dr. Robert and Laurel Adams
George and Jetta Allison
Ethan D. Alyea
Victor Anderson
Dr. Bill and Janet Anderson

Hans and Sandra Anderson
Lenore Anderson
Philip and Bonnie Clepp Anderson
Ralph and Mary Anderson
Ruth and George Asdell
Ronald P. Austin

Dave and Terry Baer

Matthew Bailey

Larry and Patti Bailey

Susanne P. Bair

Beverly C. Baker

Estate of Opal Dale Baker

Dr. Jamie Bales and Matthew Balla

Jason and Karen Banach

Jon and Brooke Barada Family

Mark and Heather Barkley

Fred M. Barrett

Janet Barrows

Lillian and David Bartlett

Patricia M. Bartlett

Dr. Mark and Mary Clare Bauman

Charles Beasley

James Becker and Anna Ochoa-Becker

Fleurette and William Benckart

Hank and Stacey Berman

Dr. Mike and Vonora Bishop

George and Jane Bloom

Bloomington High School North

Brad and Rita Bomba

Sue Huffman Bond

James H. Booze

Stephen and Carolyn M. Boyle

Mark and Katy Bradford

Dr. James Bradley and Shahla Ray

Scott and Jill Branam

Dr. Judson L. Brewer and Dr. Rebecca B. Brewer

James and Anne Bright

Philip C. Brittain

Tim and Terri Brown

E. B. Bryan

Nancy W. Bryan

Mr. John and Dr. Paula Bunde

Bruce A. Burch

Dr. Tim and Flavia Burrell

Jane B. Butcher

Stanley H. Byram Trust

Dr. David and Margery Byrne

Ernest Campaigne

Jean Campaigne

Marcia J. Campbell

Nancy and John Carlstedt

Estate of Marvin Carmack

Lucy Carmichael

Lee and Belinda Carmichael

Estate of Donald F. Carmony

The Caulfield Family

Luanne Chamness

D. L. Chatham

Phyllis and Terry Clapacs

Wanda and Robert Clegg

Dr. and Mr. M. Conger

Mark D. Conlin

D. Dale Conrad

William A. Cook

Jason Cox

Lynn and Ute Coyne

Brenda and Mike Craig

Dr. Earl and Ronda Craig

Mark and Eileen Crain

Dr. Jean and Donna Creek

Dr. William and Patricia Cron

Barbara and James Crowe

Dr. Jack A. Cummings and Dr. Marcia J. Campbell

M. Joan L. Cummins

Julie and Cary Curry

Charlie and Juli Curtis

C. Larry and Susan Davis

John F. and Melissa Davis

Harry G. Day Irrevocable Trust

Dough and DeeDee Dayhoff

Tim and Cheri DeBruicker

Estate of Charles D. DeBruler

Steve and Pam Deckard

Jack and Lisa Deinlein

Dr. Dale Dellacqua and Dr. Lisa Dellacqua

Teresa deMatas

Devin and Sandy DeWeese

Ruth C. DeWitt

Louise Dillman

Michael and Julie Donham

Vionia "Vi" Dorsett

Duke and Melinda Doster

Estate of Kathleen Dugdale

Dr. Russell and Susan Dukes

David and Jane Dunatchik

M. Tim Dunfee, MD, and Mary Ann Dunfee, RN

Charles "Pete" and Barbara Dunn

Dr. Allen and Susan Dunn

Deborah Dunn Dixon

John and Adele Edgeworth

Jean Eelma

James and Jannette W. Elliott

Dorothy and Tim Ellis

Pat and Meryl Englander

David B. Estes

Sally and Herb Fairfield

Dr. Jim and Jackie Faris

Gene and Betty Faris

Patsy Fell-Barker and Bob Barker

Pam and Kurt Felts

Theodore J. Ferguson

Dr. James and Joan Ferguson

Stephen and Connie Ferguson

John R. Figg

Mark and Jennifer Fisher

Marc and Joni Fishman

Dr. Mark and Jennifer Floyd

Victoria Franck

Carol and Joe Franklin

Dr. Heather and Karl Franklin

Carolyn and Bill Franzmann

Chuck W. Franz

Dorothy J. Frapwell

Helen T. Freeman

Ted and Kathleen Frick

Ann and Bruce Furr

Lance and Jamie Furr

Jim and Tania Gardner

Joe and Erica Garman

Donald and Carol Geels

Beth and Tony Gerth

Dr. Gary Gettelfinger

Ed and Donna Getts Sr.

Paul and Carol Gillard

John and Dana Goode

Greg and Chris Gould

James N. Grandorf

Peggy Thomas McIntire Graves

Tedd and Tara Green

David E. Greene and Barbara J. Bealer

Estate of Margaret C. Gregory

John and Rita Grunwald

Mark Guffey

Estate of Marcia Mee Guravich Hoadley

Phyllis Hackler

Richard L. Hackler

John and Cindy Hackworthy

Souheil F. Haddad

Dr. Fadi Haddad and Dr. Aline Hamati

Dr. Rajih and Darlene Haddawi

Wayne F. Hall

Donald H. Hansen

P. J. Harrah

Charles E. Harrell

Skip and Kay Beth Harrell

Dr. David and Rochelle Hart

Richard "Dick" Hasler

F. Michael Hatfield

Estate of M. Phil Hathaway

M. Phil and Margaret Hathaway

John Haury

Lois Heiser

Estate of Charles and Dorothy Heiser

Chip and Cyrilla Helm

Alisa L. Hendrix

Dr. Carter and Kate Henrich

Tom Herbert and Kirsten Roberts

Roger and Cindy Herrington

Dr. Greg Heumann and Dr. Lourdes Heumann

Karen and Bill Hicks

Estate of Art and Wilma Hill

Margaret C. Hill

Tom Hirons and Julia Riordan

Estate of Jane Hitchcock

Timothy M. Hodges, MD

George Frank Holland

Ruth Ann Holman

Estate of Stuart "Torchy" Holmquest

P. Stuart and Ann Holmquest

Dr. Paul and Marcella Holtzman

Ron and Mary Hoskins

Mary A. Howard

Estate of Mabeth Howard

Mr. Jason and Dr. Mary Howard

Rebecca Johnloz Howard

Dr. Frank and Becky Hrisomalos

Dr. Tom and Debbie Hrisomalos

Ed and Debbie Hudelson

Estate Margaret Huncilman

Estate of Robert Huncilman

Michael and Ann Hunckler

John and Christina Hurlow

Jerry M. Jesseph

Ginny and Doug Jewell

Paul and Heather Johnson

Dr. Carolyn K. Jones

Dr. Jacqueline Joyce and Dr. David Joyce

Estate of Louise Kaiser

Miles and Marjorie Kanne

Peter A. and Wanda D. Katinszky

Dr and Mrs. Jason Kennard

Dr. Bharati and Ravi Kharkar

Shapour Khosravipour, MHS, MT (ASCP)

Louise King

Paula J. Kirkman-Marlett

Buck and Andra Klemkosky

Dr. Harry Koeppen

Roland and Jan Kohr

Julius E. Krueger

Dr. Jim and Evelyn LaFollette

Dr. Vincent and Mary Lang

Charlie and Jen Laughlin

Dr. James and Catherine Laughlin

Kathie and Jim Lazerwitz

Dr. Anne M. Leach

Sara and Robert LeBien

Dr. David Y. Lee

John and Vicky Lee

Deborah Lemon

Dr. Dean Lenz

Myron D. Lewis

Dr. David Licini and Dr. Alison Heidt

Lance and Karen Like

Dr. James and Carolyn Lindsay

David and Phyllis Little

Dr. Dan and Beth Lodge-Rigal

Jane Lucas

Dr. Brandt and Dian Ludlow

Keith and Kitra Ludlow

Al and Susan Lyons

Marian Mack

P. A. Mack Jr.

Dr. Tom and Terri Madden

Dr. Mary Mahern and Dr. Clark Brittain

Dr. Richard K. Malone

E. Mayer Maloney

Harold and Alice Manifold

Lee and Annie Marchant

Edley W. Martin

Dr. Glenn and Diamond Mather

Dr. Lawrence and Jennifer McBride

Darby A. McCarty

Dr. Charles and Julia McClary

Estate of Kenneth and Virginia McConnell

Dr. Debra McDaniel and Dr. Terry McDaniel

William W. McGinnis

Dennis and Beverly McGuire

Dr. Charles R. and Sharon McKeen

Dr. Lee and Maria McKinley

Mark and Julie McMath

Dr. Kathleen McTigue and Ed Hirt

Judson Mead

Dr. and Mrs. Theodore L. Megremis

Howard D. and Carolee A. Mehlinger

Michael Melby and Maire Quilter

Rick and Mona Mellinger

Johanna Mendel

Robert F. Merchen

Don and Sonna Merk

Lee Ann Merry

R. Keith and Marion Michael

Dr. John and Gerry Miller

Ben and Christine Mitchell

Chris and Kelly Molloy

Monroe County

Stephen G. Moore

Dr. Scot Moore and Dr. Ann Moore

Kevin and Theresa Moore

Mark and Carol Moore

Dawn Morley

Wayne and Ruth Ann Morris

Thomas and Kathryn Morrison

Lyle and Irene Morton

Pat and Jack Mulholland

Richard F. Mull

Eric and Aimee Mungle

Dennis and Kristy Murphy

Estate of Walter Murphy

Jim and Rita Myers

Jean K. Nakahnikian

Jerry and Melinda Neely

Dr. Brechin and William Newby III

Roland and Carol Nobis

Estate of Lee and Deborah Norvelle

Dr. Kenneth and Mary Oglesby

Joan and Lloyd Olcott

Bill and Kathleen Oliver

Bill and Mary Oliver

Richard and Treva Olson

Lexi Orfanos

David and Sharon Ormstedt

Dan Osen

Hal J. Palmer

Halder and Catherine Palmer Trust

Angela Parker and Bret Raper

Dr. Matt and Nancy, Megan, and Matthew II Parmenter

Lowell G. Perry

Dan and Tina Peterson

Robert and Peggy Petranoff

W. George Pinnell

Dr. Anthony and Patricia Pizzo

John and Joyce Poling

Dr. George and Janice Poolitsan

Dr. Marshall Poor

Rudy and Dorothy Pozzatti

Prof. James and Kathy Pratt

Daniel Pratter

Nur Premo

Dr. William and Barbi Pugh

Paul D. Puzzello

Robert and Ilknur Ralson

Matthew and Erin Rasche

James Bradley Ray

John and Meg Ray

Richard P. and Marilyn S. Rechter

Dr, Matthew and Elva Reeck

Estate of Mary G. Reed

Estate of Charlotte Reeves

Ron and Carol Remak

Dr. Corinna, Nicole, and Emily Repetto

Tom and Jill Henderson Replogle

Barbara Restle

The Peter and Jennifer Rhoda Family

Leigh Richey

Steven and Michele Ridge

I. Taylor and Betty P. Rieger

Estate of Dagmar K. Riley

Estate of Emma B. Riley

Dr. Larry and Ellie Rink

Michael and Judy Roberts

Michael S. Roffelsen

Virginia and David Rogers

M. Darren and Michelle Root

Janice R. Ross

Robert and Sharon Rout

Dr. Todd Rowland and Mrs. Jeanne Price

Charles and Jean Royal

Dr. Jerard and Nancy Ruff

Matt and Jenny Runnebohn

Kevin L. and Judy L. Rush

John and Pat Ryan

Linda Simon and David Sabbagh

Irving J. Saltzman

Dorothy Saltzman

Rob and Missy Santa

Dr. Richard J. and Barbara Schilling

Richard and Sue Schmalz

Dr. Chad Schultheis and Dr. Ann Marie Schultheis

Terry R. Self

Dr. Frank Shahbahrami Jr. and Carrie Shahbahrami

June G. Shane

Debora J. Shaw

Steve Sheldon

Estate of Mae M. Sherman

Sue and Winston Shindell

Gene R. Shreve

Jefferson Scott Shreve

J. William Sibbitt

Estate of J. William Sibbitt Jr.

Margaret W. Sibbitt

Curt and Judy Simic

Jason Simmonds

Dr. Amy E. Simpson

Dr. Owen and Julie Slaughter

Vernon B. Smith

Bonnie Smith

Dr. Eric and Mary Smith

Dr. Alan and Kitch Somers

Nancy Sparks

Randy and Janice Sparrow

Jeanne Speakman

Tom and Karen Spradling

Dr. Andy and Peggy Stafford

Janet Stavropoulos and Michel Molenda

Dr. John and Tina Stearley

Elizabeth A. Stebbins

Dr. Timothy and Jill Steiner

Dr. Eric C. Stevens

Margaret E. Stewart

Betty Stewart

Frank R. Stewart

Ellen Stewart and Daughters

Dr. Rob Stone and Karen Green Stone

Dr. Michael and Kathryn Stowell

Dr. John and Jackie Strobel

Estate of Nancy Stultz

Terry and Betty Sturgeon

Melva L. Sturgis

Robert and Eugenie Sullivan

Paul and Ellen Surburg

Jonathan and Wendy Surdam

Dr. Mark Sutor

Sylvan Tackitt

Estate of Judy Talley

Cynthia Templeton

Dennis and Donna Terry

Dr. Kenneth Tewel Jr. and Brenda Tewel

Kevin and Beth Theile

Allan Thornton

Susan C. Thrasher

Ray Tichenor

Kamal K. Tiwari

Dr. James and Cheryl Topolgus

Dr. Carol Touloukian and Dr. James Touloukian

Randa E. Touquan

Dr. Rhonda and Tom Trippel

Virginia and Don Tyte

Gregory and Mary Ann Valenta

Sally M. Vance

John T. and Wendy B. VanderZee

Mark P. Veldman

Ann W. Viel

Susan Voelkel

Henry E. Wahl Charitable Trust

Henry and Cecilia Wahl

David Walcoff

Steve Walcoff

Judith Walcoff

Sandy and Time Wallace

Michael and Betsy Walsh

R. Scott and Pamela Walters

Jeff and Pam Warden

Mary Louise Waters Estate

Joanna Watkins, Joshua Andrew Watkins

Peggy S. Watson

Dr. Drew Watters and Dr. Melissa Watters

Rex and Dana Watters

Lee and Wylene Watts

Charles Webb

William E. Weber

Estate of Effie Wegmiller

James and Natalie Weigand

Dr. Lisa and Don Weiler

Frieda Weingart

Elizabeth Welke

Mr. Gordon and Dr. Diane Wells

Rosemary and Jack Wentworth

Bob and Edie Wetnight

Estate of Thelma Whaley

Allen R. and Nancy B. White

Dr. J. Philip White and Dr. Barbara White

Jim and Ann Whitlatch

F. Brian Whitman

Dr. Otto and Melissa Wickstrom

Charles E. and Susan D. Wier

Guy and Evelyn Wiley

Andy and Susan Williams

Shawn and Lisa Williams

Tad Wilson

Dan Pratter and Lillette Wood

John and Lisa Wrasse

Dr. Robert and Ann Wrenn

Charles and Sonya Zeller

AWARDS

Bauman Hospice Employee Award

Betty Sturgeon Cath Lab Excellence Award

BHF Employee Excellence Award

Bob Majors Supply Chain Operations Award

Brophy Early Career Excellence in Nursing Award

C. Raymond and Patricia Bartlett Advancement of
Diabetes Care Award

Cardiovascular Recovery Nursing Excellence Award

Dr. Bharati Kharkar Radiation Oncology and Radiology Award

Dr. Owen L. Slaughter Memorial Emergency Services Award

Eleanor W. Koon Community Health Award

Eleanor W. Koon Home Health Award

Emergency Medical Transport Service Award

Glen Hall Sr. Memorial Food and Nutrition Services
Education Award

Halder and Katie Palmer Rehabilitation Services Award

Helen and Fred Barrett Oncology Education Award

Helen Freeman Education Award

Jane Tourner Curry Award

Janet and Bill Anderson Obstetrical and Neonatal Nursing
Education Award

Janet Seward Dunn Medical Education Award

Joan and Marvin Carmack Exemplary Performance in Laboratory
Services Award

Judy Talley Excellence Award (nonclinical)

Katherine Anne Riley Memorial Environmental Services Award

Laughlin Neonatology Nursing Award

Margaret C. Gregory Geriatric Care Award

Mark E. Moore Servant Leadership Award

Mary and William Oliver Dementia Care Award

Medical-Surgical Nursing Services Award

Mildred B. Kohr Excellence in Nursing Award

Myron Miller Pharmacy Education Award

Nancy Stultz Psychiatric Services Award

Neurosurgical Clinic of Bloomington
    Neuroscience Excellence Award

Noble and Louise King Critical Care Services Award

Olivia C. Puzzello Pediatric Staff Award

Orthopedics of Southern Indiana Excellence Award

Psychiatric Services Award

Respiratory Care Award

Roland E. Kohr Outstanding Leadership Award

Surgery Services Award established by Bloomington
    Anesthesiologists, PC

Surgical Tech Award

Youngblood-Patton Unit Coordinator Award

CORPORATE PARTNERS

AEI

Allen Funeral Home

Anova

Artistic Media Partners

B97/Hoosier Country

Baxter Healthcare Corporation

Bell Trace Senior Living Community

Bill C. Brown Associates

Bloomfield State Bank

Bloomington Anesthesiologists

Bloomington Pediatric Dentistry

Blue and Co., LLC

Boston Scientific

BSA Lifestructures

Bunger and Robertson

CarDon and Associates, Inc.

Carmin Parker, P.C.

Cassady Electric Contractors Inc.

CFC Properties

Clendening Johnson and Bohrer

Coghlan Orthodontics

Comfort Keepers

Commercial Services Inc.

Cook Medical

Cooler Designs

Copy Co. Office Solutions

CS Property Management

Dermatology Center of Southern Indiana

Duke Energy

Elder's Journey

FA Wilhelm

FC Tucker

First Financial

Freitag and Martoglio

German American Bank

GSF USA, Inc.

Harrell-Fish Inc.

Hearthstone/Stonecroft Health Campuses

Hilliard Lyons

HOK Group, Inc

Holden Wealth Management

Home Instead

Hurlow Wealth Management

Impact Advisors

Indiana Running Company

Innovative Financial Solutions

INTIMECO Productions

IU Credit Union

IU Health Bloomington Volunteer Auxiliary

IU Health Southern Indiana Physicians

IU School of Medicine

IU School of Nursing

IU School of Public Health

Ivy Tech Community College Bloomington

Jensen Partners

Kroger

MainSource Bank

Markey's Rental and Staging

Master Rental

Meadows Hospital

Midwest Orthotics

MSP Aviation, Inc.

Myriad Genetics, Inc.

NuMotion

Old National Bank

Old National Wealth Management

Oliver Winery

Premier Healthcare

Regency Apartments

Regency Consolidated Residential, LLC

ReMax Acclaimed

Ricoh USA

Riley Physicians

Rogers Group/Rogers Group Investments

Royal on the Eastside/Royal South Toyota

Sarkes and Mary Tarzian Foundation

Shredding Unlimited

SIHO Insurance Services

SIRA Imaging Center

Smithville

Southern Indiana Pathologists

Southern Indiana Pediatric Dentistry

St. John Associates

Stampfli and Associates

Storage Express

TASUS Corporation

Taylor Imprinted Sportswear

Tenth and College/Cedarview Management

The *Herald-Times*

Tichenor Foundation

Upland Brewing Company

WBWB and WHCC

Weddle Bros Construction Company, Inc

Wells Fargo

Williams Bros

WS Property Group

WTIU/WFIU

NAMED SPACES

Barrett Family Lounge

Cook Cardiac Catheterization Laboratory

Dr. Lawrence D. Rink Cardiovascular and Pulmonary
   Rehabilitation Center

Dr. R. Kent Moseman Orthopedics Wing

Kohr Administration Building

Olcott Cancer Center

Pete and Barbara Dunn Centennial Plaza and Hospice Sanctuary

Piano in Barrett Family Lounge

Starbuck Classroom

The Bloomington Business and Professional Women's
   Club-Named Patient Room 3506

Wegmiller Auditorium

BARB BERGGOETZ, a long-time Bloomington resident who earned two IU journalism degrees, worked as a newspaper reporter, primarily at the *IndyStar* and other Indiana and Illinois daily papers, for more than 40 years. She specialized in health and fitness, education, legal, and government coverage. She also has taught at the IU Media School and Kelley School of Business. For the past six years, she has worked as a freelance writer for various publications and media outlets, including the *Washington Post*, the Center for Public Integrity and Global Integrity in Washington DC, *Bloom* magazine, and the Indiana State Medical Association.

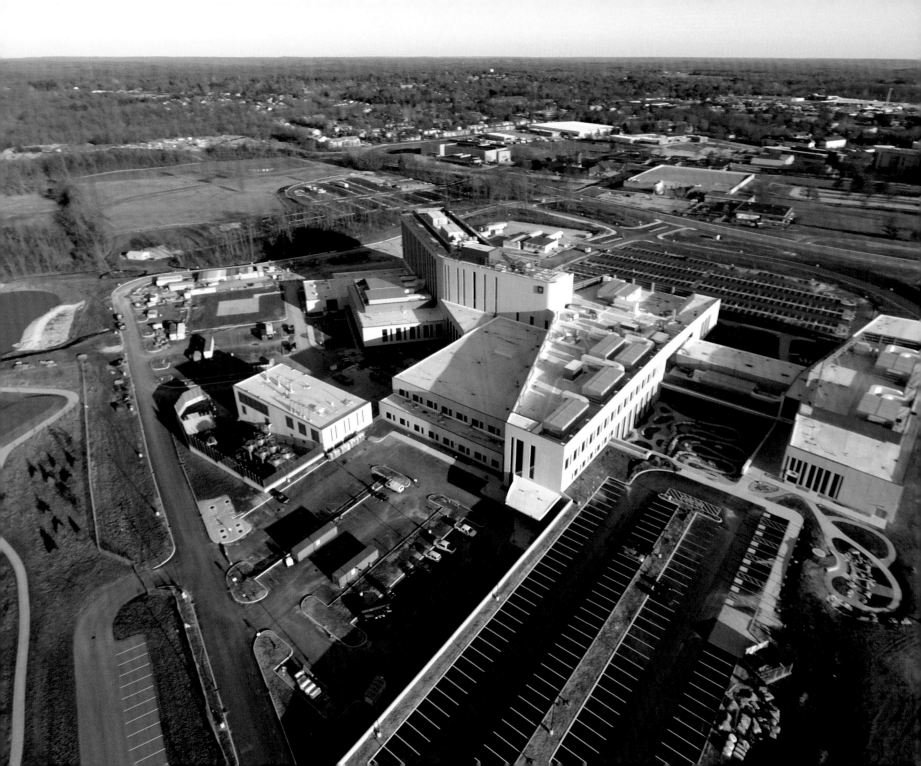